METHODS IN
MEDICAL ETHICS

Methods in Medical Ethics

Critical Perspectives

Tom Tomlinson

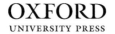

OXFORD

UNIVERSITY PRESS

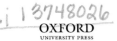

Oxford University Press, publishes works that further
Oxford University's objective of excellence
in research, scholarship, and education.

Oxford   New York
Auckland   Cape Town   Dar es Salaam   Hong Kong   Karachi
Kuala Lumpur   Madrid   Melbourne   Mexico City   Nairobi
New Delhi   Shanghai   Taipei   Toronto

With offices in
Argentina   Austria   Brazil   Chile   Czech Republic   France   Greece
Guatemala   Hungary   Italy   Japan   Poland   Portugal   Singapore
South Korea   Switzerland   Thailand   Turkey   Ukraine   Vietnam

Published by Oxford University Press, Inc.
198 Madison Avenue, New York, New York 10016
www.oup.com

Oxford is a registered trademark of Oxford University Press

Library of Congress Cataloging-in-Publication Data

Tomlinson, Thomas, 1945-
   Methods in medical ethics : critical perspectives / Tom Tomlinson.
      p. ; cm.
   Includes bibliographical references.
   ISBN 978-0-19-516124-3 (alk. paper)
   I. Title.
   [DNLM: 1. Ethics, Medical. W 50]
   LC Classification not assigned
   174.2—dc23   2011045180

9 8 7 6 5 4 3 2 1
Printed in the United States of America
on acid-free paper
Cover art by Sloan Tomlinson

To Debbie

I could never have been a philosopher without you.

ACKNOWLEDGEMENTS

I'm grateful to Jim Nelson, Hilde Lindemann, Martin Benjamin, Howard Brody, and anonymous reviewers for Oxford University Press for helpful comments on earlier versions of various chapters. They're not to blame for any nonsense that remains.

CONTENTS

INTRODUCTION

How should we set about deciding what to do when faced with an ethical problem in medicine? Is there a single best method, or is there a variety of valuable methods? And if there is a variety, are they equally useful in all the same respects? Or is each useful in some ways, but not others?

These are contentious questions, and many banners fly over this battlefield. There are camps of foundationalists, principlists, coherentists, narrativists, feminists, casuists, pragmatists, virtue theorists, care theorists, and communitarians. These divisions are fed by divergent views in moral philosophy more generally, but within medical ethics the debates have been particularly doctrinaire. There sometimes seem to be more advocates than analysts, each advocate claiming to crown the real king of ethical judgment, while laying the usurpers low.

There is certainly no dearth of bioethics literature discussing method. There are several collections of invited essays (Brody, 1988; DuBose et al., 1994; Jecker, Jonson, and Pearlman, 2007; Sugarman and Sulmasy, 2001). And there is at least one book that attempts to take a synoptic view of some parts of the controversy (Wildes, 2000). Despite the wealth of existing material, I hope this book can distinguish itself in three important ways.

First, my aim is not to declare a winner, because there is no single adequate method, as I hope to demonstrate. But neither are there any utter failures. Each method has something to add to our understanding and justification of ethical choices. This homily, found often enough in the literature, is only a milepost in the project, not its destination. The goal is to say as precisely as possible what the particular strengths and weaknesses are of each method discussed, so that by the end we have a keener idea of the sort of work each tool is best able to do. We end up with an eclecticism, but not a mindless one.

Along the way, I hope to live by two maxims. The first is to be as critical as possible of each of the methods I discuss. I embrace this maxim for several reasons. First, it is a needed corrective to the uncritical advocacy that characterizes much of the literature. Too many writers claim too much for their preferred method, and fail to acknowledge, let alone accommodate, its dangers and limits. Second, a critical gaze is the crucible that, in burning off contaminants, leaves behind whatever is of genuine value. More truth is discovered through questioning than through affirming. Of course, the danger in this approach is a negativity so curmudgeonly that it fails to see the manifest good right in front of its nose. I am by nature a skeptical person (dubbed "Doubting Thomas" by my high school biology teacher), and so suffer from this vice and must be on guard against it. I have tried to compensate for this by explicitly describing and discussing not only the limits I find in each method, but its virtues as well. The reader will decide whether I've done so fairly. Where I haven't, I aim at least to be challenging and invigorating!

My second maxim is wherever possible to illustrate whether and how theoretical criticisms of a particular method mirror real problems in medical ethics practice. This injunction too is needed as a corrective to much of the existing literature on method, which conducts the arguments at such a level of abstraction that the reader is left wondering not only how the arguments are relevant to practical ethics, but even what they are supposed to mean. This is even true, ironically, of advocacy for methods that make a special point of disparaging abstraction! It's not enough if I've made a theoretical case that a method suffers from a particular limitation; I need to show as well that the limitation raises its ugly head within the literature or practice of medical ethics, not just within the self-conscious meta-literature on method. If a problem arises only in theory, but not in practice, then it's no problem worth troubling ourselves over.

If I can be successful in these three respects, I will have some hope that this book might make a significant and lasting contribution to our understanding of methods in medical ethics.

A Word About "Method"

Depending on how the word is interpreted, the various approaches that I discuss in the chapters that follow might not all be equally understood as "methods." If method is taken to refer to an explicit set of procedures that structure our approach to a problem, then casuistry is a "method," while feminism is not, at least not always. Casuistry instructs us to use analogical reasoning to compare a problematic case with some set of less problematic cases, from which maxims may be drawn to help resolve the case. The casuist is committed to a certain structure for moral thinking, and is not partial to any particular content of the maxims employed within that structure. The feminist, by contrast, wants to draw special attention to the unfair impact of policies or practices on the less-powerful. Feminists by definition will share this goal, but employ different formal methods in pursuing it. Something similar could be said about at least some variations of virtue theory, when it emphasizes the expression of virtue over the following of rules of conduct. Like feminists, virtue theorists elevate a particular region of the moral domain for consideration, but may differ among themselves in *how* that domain is to be understood or brought to bear on particular problems.

Although neither feminism nor virtue theory is necessarily a "method" in the sense defined above, both have often been accompanied by claims of being a "method" or have been motivated by objections against some particular method, most often principle-based ones. My discussion of them pays special, although not exclusive, attention to their methodological aspirations or complaints.

If I had understood "method" differently, many other candidates could have been selected for discussion. Libertarianism and communitarianism, for example, are distinctive moral perspectives, so much so that one could say in advance what a communitarian analysis of the right to informed consent would look like, or at least what it wouldn't look like. But neither of them designates or is associated with a particular structure for moral reasoning or problem-solving[1], and so they are not included in this book.

What About Pragmatism?

In recent years, there has been an awakening of interest in the use of "pragmatist" approaches in medical ethics, reflected by the publication of several collections of essays on the topic (Keulartz et al., 2002; McGee, 1999). Yet there is not a chapter devoted to pragmatism in this book. The reason: when it comes to the pragmatic "method," there is no there there. Like John Arras (2001), I'm not convinced that a pragmatic bioethics looks or sounds distinctively different than any other approach to practical ethics.

Sometimes pragmatism is understood negatively—for example, the pragmatist is anti-foundationalist, anti-essentialist, and anti-dualist (Keulartz et al., 2002, pp. 14–15). She will take no principle or belief as absolutely true, true *a priori*, or beyond revision. Among modern scholars in moral philosophy and medical ethics, it's hard to say who's left out of this club. Within these strictures, many different approaches to moral reflection remain possible.

Other times, pragmatism is tied to the "experimental method" advocated by Peirce and extended by Dewey. The idea here is that the truth of a proposition is a matter of its success in overcoming a problematic situation, where success is judged by a community of inquirers with infinite resources and infinite time. Even if this is defensible as a conception of "true," it offers no guidance on what methods the community of inquirers can use for achieving "success." For example, it doesn't rule out the employment of moral principles that are at least provisionally taken as fixed. Dewey himself acknowledges that "Generalized ideas of ends and values undoubtedly exist. They exist not only as expressions of habit and as uncritical and probably invalid ideas, but also in the same way as valid general ideas arise in any subject. . . as tools that direct and facilitate examination of things in the concrete while they are also developed and tested by the results of their application in these cases" (*Theory of Valuation*, p. 44). In any given instance, it may be impossible to tell the pragmatist from the principlist.

The question for the pragmatists is: What will work to resolve doubt in the problematic situation? Since I hope to show that each of the methods I discuss has its uses, each of them is equally "pragmatic."

Plan of the Book

The book begins with two chapters that examine the ways in which moral principles can be employed in moral thinking.

Since the alternative methods in later chapters are all in one way or another motivated by reservations about principle-based moral reasoning, these early chapters set the stage for what follows.

The first chapter gives a sympathetic account of the lure of principles, explaining four important roles that principles play. In it, I also argue that principles are indispensable for moral thinking, despite the claims of moral particularists. In the second chapter, I defend the claim, echoed throughout the book, that although principles are indispensable, they can't be all there is to reasoned moral reflection. Using examples from two prominent bioethics scholars, I show how the interpretation and application of principles requires resort to non-principled moral resources.

Some limitations of principle-based reasoning are not shared by pluralistic moral systems, particularly when these employ a coherence model of moral justification that admits the argumentative force of specific considered judgments, not just rules and principles. The cardinal example of this is the position advocated by James Childress and Tom Beauchamp, which I discuss at length in Chapter 3. Despite the advantages I highlight, their model under-determines the moral decisions it is supposed to warrant. Such decisions require judgments of balance and interpretation that are unavoidable, but that outstrip the resources of their method.

This sets the question of whether there are any alternative modes of moral reflection that sidestep the need for such judgments, or better articulate their basis. I ask that question of the four methods taken up in the following chapters. Chapter 4 deals with casuistry. Although this is a method that looks to cases more than rules, it cannot avoid reliance on principle, nor on the judgments of interpretation and balancing that principles require. Though it is not a reliable substitute for principled reasoning, casuistry is a useful method for "ethical discovery," a notion that recurs in several of the later chapters.

Like casuistry, narrative ethics sees itself avoiding the liabilities of relying on abstract principle. Chapter 5 explores the variety of ways in which narrative can be used, concluding that "narrative coherence" is not an acceptable normative standard that can operate independently of principled moral commitments. Still, narrative tools are useful in a variety of ways, especially the uncovering of "counterstories" that help to enrich the moral considerations taken into account.

Feminist ethics, like narrative ethics, has been understood in a variety of ways, some of which are motivated by reaction against abstract moral principle. Chapter 6 is organized around three different conceptualizations of feminist ethics. Feminist concerns with the institutionalized abuse of power help remind us of important dimensions of ethical problems that are frequently overlooked. Some feminists, however, place an undue faith in attention to context, when such attention is unguided by more general commitments.

Chapter 7 examines several different sorts of virtue theory and shows that reliance on virtue cannot be a wholesale substitute for commitments to principles. Nevertheless, asking questions about virtue can open up new avenues for ethical deliberation that are pertinent for evaluating not just persons, but their actions as well.

The final chapter uses examples of three different kinds of medical ethics problems to further illustrate and compare the strengths, limits, and uses of the methods discussed in the book. The lesson is that no matter what the problem, every one of the methods might find a role to play at particular junctures in the argument, a role that makes use of that method's characteristic strengths.

A Word About Judgment

As the reader will soon discover, one pervasive theme in the book is the unavoidable need for good judgment. None of these methods succeeds at being algorithmic. No matter the method, the sorts of reasons it assembles lead with certainty to no single conclusion. Regardless how thorough, conscientious, and sophisticated the application of the method, there comes a point where one simply must decide where the balance of argument lies. Since the method has already been exhausted, that final judgment can't be warranted by the method. Sure enough, the judgment is based on the reasoning and evidence brought forward under the method. But the judgment is not determined only by a method, but by a faculty, one might say.

Or so I've come to believe in the course of writing this book. Originally, I planned to devote a chapter to characterizing this faculty, reviewing ways of developing and, if possible, even evaluating it. But I've since lost confidence that it would be possible to do this justice in a single chapter. I've even lost confidence that philosophical tools are up to the job. I suspect this explains why virtually all philosophical treatment of "moral judgment" is about the proper *grounds for* moral decisions, not about how one gets from those grounds to a *decision* about which course of action they warrant in a particular situation.

It may be that acts of judgment are at bottom performative, rather than evaluative, in the sense that Nozick had in mind when he remarked that "reasons don't come with previously given precisely specified weights; the decision process is not one of discovering such precise weights, but of assigning them" (Nozick, 1981, p. 294).

Even if reasons don't determine the judgment that needs to be made, good judgments still require good reasons. This book explores the variety of good reasons at our disposal.

Note

1 Except on occasion methods already discussed in this book. An example is Mark Kuczewski's (1997) marriage of communitarianism and casuistry.

Bibliography

Arras, John D. 2001. "Freestanding Pragmatism in Law and Bioethics." *Theoretical Medicine* 22: 69–85.

Brody, Baruch. 1988. *Moral Theory and Moral Judgments in Medical Ethics*. Dordrecht: Kluwer Academic Publishers.

DuBose, Edwin R., Ron Hamel and Laurence J. A. O'Connell. 1994. *Matter of Principles: Ferment in U.S. Bioethics*. Valley Forge, PA: Trinity Press International.

Jecker, Nancy S., Albert R. Jonson and Robert Pearlman. 2007. *Bioethics: Introduction to History, Methods, and Practice*, 2nd ed. Sudbury, MA: Jones & Bartlett.

Keulartz, Josef, Michiel Korthals, Maartje Schermer, and Tsjalling Swierstra. 2002. *Pragmatist Ethics for a Technological Culture*. Dordrecht: Kluwer Academic Publishers.

Kuczewski, Mark G. 1997. *Fragmentation and Consensus: Communitarian and Casuist Bioethics*. Washington, D.C.: Georgetown University Press.

McGee, Glenn. 1999. *Pragmatic Bioethics*. Nashville: Vanderbilt University Press.

Nozick, Robert. 1981. *Philosophical Explanations*. Cambridge: Harvard University Press.

Sugarman, Jeremy and Daniel P. Sulmasy. 2001. *Methods in Medical Ethics*. Washington, D.C.: Georgetown University Press.

Wildes, Kevin William. 2000. *Moral Acquaintances: Methodology in Bioethics*. Notre Dame: University of Notre Dame Press.

Chapter 1

The Indispensability of Principles

In this chapter and the next, I want to characterize and begin to evaluate a prevailing view of how one justifies moral judgments in medical ethics. This is the view, sometimes called "principlism," that maintains that giving reasons in ethics consists mainly—if not exclusively—in appealing to general principles or rules,[1] from which more specific moral conclusions should be derived by some form of inference.

This is not just a philosopher's unnatural fantasy. In normal moral discourse we often appeal to rules, regardless of whether we are tutored in the vocabulary of the moral philosopher:

"Unfortunately many may disagree but I believe that life, like all things are determined through random actions. Let's take an example of dice. If we roll twelve dice, they won't land all on the same side. Why, because it's all random. I believe that life is just as random, that is why people are different and handicapped, because life is random, it's different every time. Even though genetic material from the parents determine whether a person will be tall or short, there is always a possibility of having a defect, or disease. If cloning can help mankind, reduce the risks and diseases then why not clone. It's helping the odds at a better life of a new person." (Posted on a listserv discussion of cloning. Edited for spelling.)

Clearly this person believes that human cloning should be permitted, and he offers reasons for his view. Those reasons include claims about matters of fact—for example, that random genetic events influence the quality of human life, and that cloning could reduce this randomness. It also includes claims about values— for example, that the results of randomness are too often bad, and that we should reduce these bad outcomes when we have the means to do so.

Put the claims about the facts together with the claims about the values, and we have an attempt at reasoned ethical argument (despite what you may think of its quality). At the heart of the argument is a general rule about what ought to be done: a principle that tells us we should act to improve the quality of people's lives. Once we've determined that cloning can accomplish this goal, we have the elements of an argument on behalf of cloning:

1. We should act to improve the quality of people's lives when we have the means.
2. Human cloning can be used to effectively improve the quality of people's lives.
3. Therefore, we should permit human cloning.

This common form of ethical reasoning—appeals to principles or rules within a deductive form of argument—has also been attractive to moral philosophers and medical ethicists. We will want to better understand both its attractions and its problems as a form of justification.

Reasons and Rules

Let's begin that evaluation by asking why anyone would think that principles or rules are the main tool of ethical reasoning. A stock medical ethics example will help illustrate why this model is an attractive one:

Mr. Heyes is a 75-year-old man in the intensive care unit who is suffering from multiple and interrelated conditions, including congestive heart failure and renal failure. A heart attack shortly after admission led to him being intubated and placed on a ventilator. He remains stuporous and unable to communicate. His physicians believe that even though his condition is serious, options for treatment are not yet exhausted. With luck, he might recover enough to return to his home, where previously he had led a precariously independent life. His daughter (the only close surviving family member) is concerned, however, about her father's often-stated desire not to be "hooked to machines," or "be left a vegetable" who is "no good to anyone." His daughter is requesting that no further life-prolonging treatments be instituted; Mr. Heyes' physicians are opposed to this.

It has often been argued[2] that what distinguishes ethical attitudes from many other kinds of preferences is that ethical judgments call for the giving of reasons. Asking someone to defend her preference for pistachio ice cream with reasons hardly seems pertinent. By contrast, it is always pertinent to ask her to offer reasons for ethical judgments across a wide range of her attitudes concerning other-regarding actions, from her beliefs about the morality of abortion to her decision that she should lie to her best friend about where she was last night.

And so we could rightly ask both his physicians and his daughter to defend their positions regarding Mr. Heyes' treatment with reasons. What might they say?

Perhaps the daughter would argue that treatment should be limited because that is what her father would want. If someone challenged her by asking why that should matter, she might respond that doctors should never apply treatments which an adult patient would refuse. Unlike her first answer, the second one is the assertion of a rule, general enough to apply to all adult patients and all doctors, not just her father and his physicians.

One argument for the necessity of principles in ethical reasoning, then, is that principles or rules are what we end up with when we press the demand for reasons; a demand that is, at least up to a point, always legitimate to make in ethical matters.[3]

Another kind of argument on behalf of principles starts with the requirement of universalizability. If my ethical judgments are not merely arbitrary or *ad hoc*, I will concede that at least I must be consistent: I should judge all like cases alike. Indeed, the doctors caring for Mr. Heyes might point out other cases like his where they have also felt obligated to insist on continuing treatment. Surely, however, these cases weren't *exactly* like his; for instance, the patients didn't all weigh the same. They would be like one another only in certain relevant respects. Those relevant respects would be general features common to all the specific cases, which together would explain why they made the same moral judgment of them all. When pressed for an accounting of the common features among the cases they describe, the physicians might say that they are all situations in which the patient left no specific evidence regarding his wishes and in which the patient had what the physicians believed to be a significant possibility of recovery. This is as much to assert the moral rule that when an incompetent patient has left no specific evidence regarding his wishes and he still has some chance of recovery, his treatment should continue.

And so, moral principles can serve to unify or systematize our more specific moral judgments. In so doing, they offer some safeguard against capricious inconsistency of judgment. At the very least, the physicians caring for Mr. Heyes have the burden of showing that their decision in his case is not arbitrarily at odds with their judgments in other cases, and an appeal to principle is the means by which this burden is met. Principles supply a medium through which our various moral beliefs are related to one another, making it possible to use some of our moral beliefs to critically evaluate other moral beliefs. Mr. Heyes' daughter may be able to describe a set of circumstances in which a family member's testimony with respect to the patient's wishes is trustworthy, despite the lack of direct evidence from the patient. Would the physicians agree that in those circumstances they should respect the family member's choices, out of respect for their duty not to use interventions that the patient would refuse? If so, then they would have a principled reason to revise their rule, and perhaps their judgment of what to do with Mr. Heyes.

Third, to think of moral reasoning as relying on rules or principles allows us to keep it within a more general and well-understood model of reasoning: deductive inference. If Mr. Heyes' daughter were of a systematic frame of mind, she might schematize her reasoning like this:

A. Doctors should never apply treatments that an adult patient would refuse.
B. Mr. Heyes (my father) would refuse further treatment for his condition.
C. (Therefore) His doctors should not apply any further treatment for his condition.

In its logical structure, this is no different than the trite syllogism:

A' All men are mortal.
B' Socrates is a man.
C' (Therefore) Socrates is mortal.

Granting the truth of the premises, the conclusion follows with a certainty in either case. If ethical reasoning—or some parts of it—are deductive in character, such reasoning is not only clear and familiar, but it also focuses our attention on critical questions in a straightforward way. In common moral discourse, reason-giving is elliptical. Hidden assumptions need to be made explicit. Thinking of ethical argument as at least partly deductive in form provides a framework that makes it possible to specify premises that are otherwise only implicitly assumed. As we fill in these additional premises, we can recognize where the argument requires additional evidence to support those premises, and we can sharpen our understanding of the roots of ethical disagreement. Once Mr. Heyes' daughter makes the minor premise explicit, for example, we will recognize how critical it will be to establish what Mr. Heyes' would have in fact refused. To the extent that the premise is contestable, so will be the ethical conclusion that it supports.

Fourth, something like principles seem to form the content of our moral sensibility, functioning as "rules of moral salience," in Barbara Herman's phrase. They serve to identify morally relevant features of the environment, alerting us to the possibility that we are entering morally risky territory that may require us to make a moral judgment. If it weren't for our knowledge of rules like "Pay heed to persons' wishes regarding their own lives," "Avoid doing harmful things to others," and "Save life when possible," neither Mr. Heyes' daughter nor his physicians would have any sense that his care presented a moral question at all. Principles in this role don't tell us what we should do. Rather, they direct our attention to the sorts of things that must be taken into account in deciding on the ethically appropriate course of action. Thus, principles play an essential role in the beginning of deliberation, and not only toward its end.

So there are four reasons one might suppose that principles are indispensable for ethical reasoning. They are where the demand for reasons leads us; they provide a medium for systematizing and critically evaluating our ethical beliefs; they enable ethical reasoning to be characterized as a form of deductive inference, which in turn supplies useful tools of analysis and critique; and they direct our attention to the morally relevant features of the situations we face.

Must Reasons Be Rules?

Considerations such as these show that moral principles, and deductive arguments employing them, are useful, perhaps even indispensable, elements in moral discourse. But this claim should not be confused with a much stronger one: That reasons in ethics *must always* take the form of rules.

None of the virtues of principles described above would support this claim. First, the fact that ethical inquiry demands *reasons* says nothing about what form those reasons must take. Certainly, the reasons that people offer may often take the form of general principles figuring in a deductive argument. But without some further inquiry, it would beg the question to assume that reasons in ethics *can be* of no other sort. The question of what forms reasoned reflection could take in ethics can be answered only by characterizing and evaluating the sorts of considerations other than appeals to principle that people in fact offer in support of their moral views. That will be the primary objective of several chapters to follow.

If other sorts of reasons are possible, then we may also be able to systematize and critique our moral beliefs without always making use of principles or rules. This would require the use of forms of inference beside deduction, or the legitimation of non-inferential forms of moral knowledge. It may well be that thinking of ethical arguments as deductive in form is often advantageous. This observation is, however, perfectly compatible with the assertion that it is sometimes disadvantageous to think of ethical argument in this way, or that there are advantages to considering alternative forms of moral knowledge and reflection.

Finally, even if we agree with Herman that rules of moral salience structure our moral sensibility, it wouldn't follow that rules govern our reasoned judgments of how to best accommodate the moral considerations to which our attention had been drawn. Knowing what must be considered, and reasoning how to respond to those considerations, may be two different matters.

Universalizability and Rules

There is nevertheless an argument that has frequently been made in support of the strong claim that moral reasons must be rules. The most widely known version of the argument is made by R.M. Hare,[4] but it has also been deployed more recently by writers in medical ethics.[5] As a simple requirement of consistency, Hare tells us, it follows from any particular moral judgment that some more general moral judgment or principle must be assumed to be true. If I say of one action that it is "right," but refuse to call "right" a second action that I admit is exactly like the first, then I am inconsistent. "This is right," then, implies "Everything exactly like this in every respect is right." Now since no two things are *exactly* alike, we may safely say that:

(a) "*This is right*" implies "*Everything like this in relevant respects is right.*"

This has not yet given us a "principle" properly so called, Hare goes on, since it contains the individuating term "this." But we may readily eliminate this term by specifying what the "relevant respects" are, which yields the universal principle:

(b) *Everything with features a... n is right.*

One might object straightaway that we know of no unexceptionable principles that would take this form. To date, it might be claimed that any proposed principles have been refuted with counter-examples, and so as a matter of experience we should conclude that there are no unexceptionable principles.

But this objection does not touch Hare's conclusion, for Hare's argument is an *a priori* one purporting to show that such principles *must* exist, as a matter of logical necessity. It will hardly do to argue against this from the merely *a posteriori* claim that as a matter of fact we have not yet discovered them, for Hare's argument is designed to prove that they exist nonetheless, even if, as Hare admits, it may be a matter of the most difficult sort specifying what the "relevant respects" are.

In fact, though, Hare's argument fails for a more fundamental reason. Note that strictly speaking, the inference in (a) is not one required by consistency. Consistency in making the claim "This is right" requires only the admission that "Everything exactly like this is right." There is nothing inconsistent in saying of two actions that they are alike in all other respects, except that one is "right," and the other not. These judgments do not imply any statement of the form "Action A is both right and not-right," unless "right" is defined naturalistically, to literally *mean* "has properties a... n."

Of course, one need not be a naturalist to think that moral "properties" are, in Moore's expression, "supervenient"— that is, their ascription depends upon the presence of non-moral properties of actions and states of affairs.[6] But this claim regarding supervenience has always seemed to me (and I will not argue for it here) to be nothing more than the assertion that moral language is inherently rational—if I make a moral judgment, I must be prepared to give reasons that refer to some properties possessed by that which is judged. It is *together with* the assumption that moral language is rational that different moral judgments about otherwise similar acts become inconsistent, since whatever reason I would offer for calling the one "right" would apply with equal force to the other.

It is this assumption, then, that authorizes the inference in (a) to "everything like this in relevant respects is right," for a property is "relevant," after all, precisely because it constitutes a reason for calling a thing "right." The consequent in (a) may now be translated to "everything of which I may affirm the same reasons as my reasons for calling this right, is also right."

The abstract principle (b) then becomes:

(b')Everything to which reasons A. . . N apply is right.

The appeal to universalizability, remember, is supposed to prove that any particular judgment of rightness relies upon a substantive moral principle of the form "All so-and-so's are right." But once we have determined what (b) means, we no longer have as our conclusion a schema for a moral principle. (b') is silent on the question of what sorts of propositions are to count as the reasons for making the judgment—they may take the form of constitutive principles, but (b') does not require that they do. So far as the requirement of universalizability is concerned, these reasons might take the form of a story, or an analogy with a case, or one of the other forms of ethical reflection to be discussed in this book.

The principle of universalizability should not have been expected to support any conclusion about the role of constitutive principles in ethical justification. The principle, after all, is simply a statement of the idea that any rational system requires the consistent application of reasons, a requirement that applies to any mode of reasoning, whatever its form or content. The question of constitutive principles is not a question about consistency. What we want to know about principles is not "If we use principles as the only court of appeal in moral reasoning, should we use them wherever applicable?" That would be quite pointless to ask. Rather, what we want to know is whether it is principles only that provide the reasons for moral judgments.

Hare's argument demonstrates the necessity of constitutive moral principles only on the *assumption* that moral reasoning is exclusively deductive. Once that assumption is made, of course, it follows without further argument that universal principles are the evidence on which our moral conclusions must rest, and that principles are the only reasons to which one may appeal.

This argument, then, along with variations on it (e.g., Frankena, pp. 24–25), shows neither that moral argument requires constitutive principles, nor that it is necessarily or exclusively deductive in form.[7]

Reasons Can't Be Rules?

We've just considered, and rejected, the strong claim that reasons in ethics can only consist of rules. We must now turn attention to an equally strong claim at the opposite end of the spectrum: that reasons can't be matters of rules, because there can be no rules.

This is the position that has come to be known as "particularism," and is associated with the work of philosophers like John McDowell and Jonathan Dancy. "The leading thought behind particularism," Dancy says, "is the thought that the behaviour of a reason (or of a consideration that serves as a reason) in a new case cannot be predicted from its behaviour elsewhere... so there is no ground for the hope that we can find out here how that consideration functions *in general*" (Dancy, p. 60). If a moral principle is understood to identify a general consideration that offers a reason either for or against an action, then, there can be no moral principles.

Reasons in ethics don't function in this way, Dancy argues, because moral considerations interact with one another in particular circumstances in unpredictable ways. In some circumstances, a particular factor will count as a reason in favor of an action; in other circumstances, it will count against; and in yet others it won't matter at all.

He gives a number of examples intended to illustrate this "holism" of moral reasons. For example:

> "I borrow a book from you, and then discover that you have stolen it from the library. Normally, the fact that I have borrowed the book from you would be a reason to return it to you, but in this situation it is not. It isn't that I have *some* reason to return it to you and more reason to put it back in the library. I have no reason at all to return it to you."
>
> (Dancy, p. 61)

And so, there can be no principle like "One should return what's borrowed" that could reliably function as a reason entering into our deliberation about what to do.

Dancy thinks that similar examples can be constructed around any proffered moral principle or rule. It's easy enough to imagine examples from health care ethics in which a factor switches its "moral valence." Ordinarily, the fact that a patient has signed a consent form is a reason that favors proceeding with treatment. But if the patient's signature was manipulated or coerced, it doesn't morally count at all.

We should first ask whether such examples support Dancy's radical conclusion. Take the borrowed book. Hasn't Dancy simply failed to uncover the principle really at work? It may well be that the principle that I should return what is borrowed is particular to the circumstances, but how about the principle that I should return what belongs to another? Such a principle explains the moral valence of "being borrowed" both in ordinary circumstances and in the situation that Dancy describes, since there the book belongs to the library, not my friend. The deeper moral consideration is not "being borrowed;" it's "being owed."

We can make similar observations about "having signed a consent form." This is of superficial moral relevance. Its relevance is a function of something deeper, like "having the patient's permission." The former factor has switched its moral valence between the two circumstances; the latter has not.

The problem here, as Roger Crisp explains in his discussion of Dancy's examples, is that Dancy fails to distinguish between "ultimate" and "non-ultimate" reasons (see Crisp, pp. 36ff). We don't have to embrace Crisp's terminology to appreciate the point that when operating with superficial moral reasons, one shouldn't be surprised to see them operating differently in different circumstances. Our explanation of such phenomena will rely upon a deeper or more general moral claim.

With respect to these, it becomes much harder to devise counterexamples in which the more basic reason switches its valence. What one ends up with instead are examples in which basic reasons are in conflict with one another, and some judgment is called for in deciding what to do. What should I do when my friend, who has given me his weapon for safekeeping, demands its return when he is in a murderous rage? (Socrates' example in Plato's *Republic*). What if a patient has freely requested a treatment that I believe is more harmful than beneficial? But such examples show only that a moral reason that is decisive in some situations is not decisive in others, not that the reason doesn't count at all, or counts in an entirely different way. This is a phenomenon that is compatible with the use of general moral principles.

As Crisp points out, an act utilitarian, who has as her ultimate principle the requirement to take that action that produces the greatest aggregate good, can both advocate the adoption of subsidiary principles (like "Respect patient choices") and explain why in some particular circumstance that subsidiary principle should not be decisive (see Crisp, p. 32). The same sort of thing can be said of a moral theory like Ross', which accepts that there are a number of moral principles ("Don't lie;" "Do good"). In morally complex situations these may come into conflict, and we have to decide how these conflicting commitments are to be negotiated or resolved. This judgment may not itself be a direct inference from a rule, and so may require the employment of something beyond the principles involved. But the fact that the principles aren't *all* there is to our moral reflection doesn't mean that they play no important role at all.

Dancy calls this sort of particularism—in which the decisiveness of a moral principle or set of principles is particular to the circumstance of its application—a "particularism of rules," and distinguishes it from the more radical particularism he wants to defend (Dancy, p. 56). But this is the weaker position toward which he is driven under critical examination of his examples.

This is because there is a deeper problem for particularism: how to preserve a plausible account of moral reasoning. Dancy wants to claim that reasons are particular, not that reasons are not possible in ethics. But can reasons be so radically particular as Dancy claims, and remain reasons of any sort?

Why should the fact that you have stolen the book from the library nullify the moral relevance of my having borrowed it? Dancy agrees that the particularist, like any other moralist, is bound to give reasons for his moral claims. What would these look like? Sometimes, Dancy's holism of reasons suggests that all I can do is point to the same facts for which an explanation is being sought. Why did my having borrowed the book not matter? Because it was stolen.

Now it's true that often all that's required is that some particular feature of the situation be brought to light for us to understand why it is that we should respond differently than we would in other circumstances. Pointing to that particular new feature is not yet to make any claim about its relevance in other circumstances, but it may be enough to lead you to see the moral situation in the same way I do.

It won't be enough, however, if you *aren't* led to see the moral situation the same as I, if instead you ask why the new feature should make the difference I claim it does. If all I can do is point once more to that particular configuration of factors, then I've run out of reasons. I can only hope that by dint of insistent repetition it will get through your thick skull.

If instead I take your question more seriously, the reasons I offer will have to make some reference to generalizations—principles by which this particular set of circumstances, and the moral pertinence of the feature in question, is set into a larger context that explains why the feature should have the effect that I claim it does. As I've just admitted, not all explanations require appeal to some larger framework. Sometimes it's enough to just point. But, just as importantly, sometimes it's not.

If appeal to some level of generalization is a critical element of explanation in complex or contested matters, we shouldn't be surprised to find Dancy making use of general principles. For example:

> "It seems that the way in which pleasure and fun function as reasons is logically dependent on the nature of the activity we are enjoying. Consider the suggestion that we have more reason to have public executions of convicted rapists if the event would give pleasure both to the executioner and to the crowds that would no doubt attend. Surely this pleasure is a reason against rather than a reason for"
>
> (Dancy, p. 61)

Unlike his other examples, here Dancy has given himself an interlocutor who's offered the suggested case. In the face of a potential disputant, Dancy can't rest content with merely asserting its contrary, and so he must complete the sentence with a reason: "pleasure at a wrong action compounds the wrong." Of course, this is a statement of general principle, which to be persuasive must be making implicit appeal to other circumstances in which we would agree that this is true. Its use assumes that the judgments made there are relevant to the judgment we should make here. This is a generalist assumption.

The presence of an interlocutor is significant, because it underscores the importance of the argumentative situation. We can afford to be radically particularist about reasons when contemplating situations in which moral judgment is unproblematic. But when confronted by uncertainty, in the form either of our internal ambivalence or the disagreement of others, further understanding of the dimensions of that uncertainty, let alone any resolution of it, will not always be found entirely within the very situation that has caused the uncertainty.

The failure to take account of the argumentative situation infects Dancy's discussion of forms of argument that attempt to draw conclusions about the moral relevance of a feature in one situation by making inferences from its relevance in another situation. The example he uses to illustrate this mode of reasoning is a famous analogy used by James Rachels. Rachels argues against the traditional distinction made between active and passive euthanasia, embodied in the American Medical Association's position that "mercy killing" is absolutely prohibited, while the withdrawal of "extraordinary means" that "lets the patient die" is permissible. Rachels offers several arguments against this doctrine, but one in particular employs an analogy. Imagine two men, both of whom plot the death of their six-year-old cousin in order to inherit his fortune. The one man, Smith, slips into the bathroom and drowns the child as he's taking his bath. The other man, Jones, also enters the bathroom, but as he does, the child slips in the tub and is knocked unconscious. Jones then merely stands by and watches his cousin drown. Rachels takes it that what Smith does is an active "killing" and what Jones does is a passive "letting die;" but both acts are equally wrong. The conclusion Rachels draws is that "the bare difference between killing and letting die does not, in itself, make a moral difference" (Rachels, 1975, p. 79).

Dancy takes Rachels to be arguing that the distinction between killing and letting die "is not morally relevant anywhere" (Dancy, p. 89) since it is not morally relevant in the case of Smith and Jones. This is exactly the sort of universal claim that a particularist rejects, which is what Dancy does. He offers a contrasting case: Imagine being forced to choose between allowing two children to die, or killing one. Clearly, Dancy says, it would be worse to kill the one, even if thereby more children die. In *these* circumstances, the distinction between killing and letting die is morally relevant. Since the relevance of the distinction is utterly context-dependent, Rachels can't use its irrelevance in the Smith–Jones case to draw any conclusions about its relevance for end-of-life care.

This ignores the argumentative situation in which Rachels deploys his analogy. The analogy is a response to the claim that the AMA doctrine is justified *because* killing is morally worse than letting die. To challenge this argument, Rachels doesn't have to make the claim that Dancy attributes to him—that no matter what the circumstances, killing is never worse than letting die. (Indeed, elsewhere in the article he offers explanations for why killing is usually worse than letting die.) All his analogy needs to do is impose a burden of proof on those who, in the face of demands for reasons, fall back on the distinction to explain why it offers a sound argument in favor of the AMA doctrine.

But even this more modest purpose, which seems essential to the conduct of reasoned discourse, is out of bounds for Dancy. The Smith–Jones example establishes that the distinction doesn't always matter. This much is perfectly compatible with Dancy's particularism. It's the next step that Dancy can't take: that therefore, those who use the distinction to defend the AMA doctrine need to explain why it's relevant here. If radical particularism is true, the relevance of a reason in one situation has nothing to do with its relevance in another, and can't impose any burden of proof.

What, then, would be left for someone like Rachels who is not persuaded by the reasons offered by defenders of the AMA doctrine? Sullen silence, it would seem. Unable to draw on any moral principles or cases that lie outside the boundaries of the disputed situation, he is left with no tools by which to challenge, and through which to engage with, those with whom he disagrees. This is the stark consequence of a radical particularism of reasons. Its unacceptability suggests the vital role that appeals to general, if not absolute, moral claims must play in making reasoned moral discourse possible.

Principles: Neither All nor Nothing

We are led, then, to reject two strong claims about the role of principles in moral reasoning. On the one hand, it remains to be shown that ethical reasons can only take the form of principles or rules. The principle of universalizability requires that our moral judgments be consistently based in reasons, but it doesn't dictate the form those reasons must take. On the other hand, our reasons can't be utterly particular to each situation in a way that abjures all use of moral principles. Especially in situations of moral disagreement, we must have some recourse to general moral claims in order to develop deeper levels of critical moral understanding and justification. Principles can play important roles in moral discourse, and aren't to be lightly cast aside.

These conclusions leave two questions open. First, are principles alone adequate to explaining and justifying our moral judgments? If not, in what particular ways are they not enough? And second, what non-principled modes of moral reflection are there? Are they able to substitute for principles, or are they complementary to them, compensating for the inadequacies of principles alone? These are the questions I begin to pursue in the next chapter.

Notes

1. In these chapters, I will use "principles" and "rules" interchangeably. Although rules are sometimes distinguished from principles as being more specific and concrete, this is not a distinction that bears on my discussion.

2. For example, see Toulmin, 1970, Section 4–4.

3. See Toulmin, p. 146. The philosophical imperative is to push the "Why?" question to its limits, which leads to the development of a normative moral theory.

4. The version of the argument that I discuss is found in Section 2.2 of Hare's *Freedom and Reason* (Hare, 1963). In his later work, Hare does not repeat this argument in so compact a form, but he clearly relies on the idea that the principle of universalizability mandates reliance on general principles to supply the justification for moral judgments, even if these principles can be known only by an "archangel." See, for

example, Section 6.4 of *Moral Thinking* (Hare, 1981), as well as his entry in the *Encyclopedia of Ethics* (Hare, 1992).

5. See for example, Beauchamp and Childress, 4th ed., p. 26. This appeal to universalizability disappeared from the 5th edition.

6. See "The Conception of Intrinsic Value," reprinted in the revised edition of *Principia Ethica*, pp. 280–298.

7. The preceding discussion of Hare is drawn from Tomlinson, 1980, Chapter 2.

Bibliography

Brink, David O. 1989. *Moral Realism and the Foundations of Ethics.* New York: Cambridge University Press.

Crisp, Roger. 2000. "Particularizing Particularism." In Hooker and Little, op. cit., pp. 23–47.

Dancy, Jonathan. 1993. *Moral Reasons.* Oxford: Blackwell.

Frankena, William K. 1973. *Ethics*, 2nd ed. Englewood Cliffs, NJ: Prentice-Hall.

Hare, R.M. 1963. *Freedom and Reason.* London: Oxford University Press.

Hare, R.M. 1981. *Moral Thinking.* New York: Oxford University Press.

Hare, R.M. 1992. "Universalizability." In *Encyclopedia of Ethics*, ed. Lawrence C. and Charlotte B. Becker. New York: Garland Publishing.

Herman, Barbara. 1993. "The Practice of Moral Judgment." In Barbara Herman, *The Practice of Moral Judgment*. Cambridge, MA: Harvard University Press: 73–93.

Hooker, Brad, and Margaret Little. 2000. *Moral Particularism.* New York: Oxford.

Larmore, Charles E. 1987. *Patterns of Moral Complexity.* New York: Cambridge University Press.

Moore, G.E. 1993. *Principia Ethica.* Revised edition with "Preface to the second edition" and other papers, ed. T. Baldwin, Cambridge: Cambridge University Press.

Rachels, James. 1975. "Active and Passive Euthanasia." *New England Journal of Medicine* 292 (2): 78–80.

Rachels, James. 1993. *The Elements of Moral Philosophy*, 2nd ed. New York: McGraw-Hill.

Ross, W.D. 1939. *The Foundations of Ethics*. Oxford: Oxford University Press.

Tomlinson, Thomas. 1980. *The Use of Principles in Moral Reasoning*. E. Lansing: Michigan State University (unpublished dissertation).

Toulmin, Stephen. 1970. *Reason in Ethics*. London: Cambridge University Press.

Chapter 2

The Limits of Principles

The principle of universalizability has not shown that our ethical reasoning must always employ principles. The particularist has not shown that our ethical reasoning can never employ general principles. Principles may remain pragmatically indispensable to reasoned moral discourse, even if not logically necessary. But even if essential, they may alone be inadequate, requiring the employment of other modes of moral reflection. Are principles alone adequate to the task of justifying our moral attitudes? Most of the criticism that has been leveled in recent years against "principlism" or "deductivism" has purported to show that they are not. These are the criticisms to which I will now turn.

There are only a couple of basic critical strategies available for challenging the adequacy of principles, although each of these permits some number of variations.

There Is No Conclusive Agreement on a Normative Theory

The first strategy is to question the theoretical warrant for any principle that might be offered as justification for a moral conclusion. For a systematic normative theory like utilitarianism or Kantianism, one might criticize the philosophical arguments undergirding the principle of utility, or the categorical imperative. Armies of moral philosophers have mined this approach for generations, to no well-accepted conclusion. This fact itself has been used as an argument against reliance on principles in medical ethics. Arthur Caplan, in one of the earliest attacks on principlism, notes that "Questions about the moral standing of the comatose, the senile, or the retarded may require recourse to the concepts of moral philosophy, but no single moral theory has, or claims to provide, a definitive answer for the proper treatment and care that ought to be given to individuals in these categories." This is in part because "In many problem areas, no *single* moral theory can lay claim to the mantle of truth" (Caplan, 1980, p. 27; italics his).

This is a genuine problem only for a *monistic* normative theory. A monistic system aspires to ground moral justification in a single principle, or in a small set of hierarchically ordered principles. These think of moral justification on the model of geometry, in which a set of given axioms generates a system of more specific principles, which are in turn applied to the facts provided by particular circumstances, whether the facts be geometric or ethical. The exemplar is utilitarianism, which has as its guiding principle to maximize the good. All further rules and decisions are to be based, directly or indirectly, on this single principle.[1] If that single principle is called into question, so is the whole system.

A *pluralistic* system disavows any interest in or need for an overarching normative theory that provides a final justification for its principles, and on which the whole system stands or falls.[2] A pluralistic system employs some number of principles as starting points for moral justification. These may be principles taken to be intuitively obvious to any person of moral sense, or so deeply entrenched within a culture as to be unquestionable. The principles are unordered, each making its independent demand on us. So long as there is agreement about the set of basic principles, there is no need to provide some further justification for them, since none is called for. To cast doubt on the usefulness of principles, one would have to reject the whole lot, not a very plausible strategy.

Although pluralistic systems may avoid the first objection to the use of principles, they remain vulnerable to other problems.

There Is Insoluble Conflict Between Principles

Pluralistic systems may avoid becoming ensnared in disputes about foundational theories only to face their own characteristic problem: how to resolve conflicts among principles. Since conflicts between basic norms may be a necessary feature of moral life (see Kekes, 1993), any pluralistic system must offer some account of how to respond to these conflicts in a reasoned way that will support a chosen course of action. A monistic system like utilitarianism has in theory a way to handle these, since the foundational or overarching principle is intended to provide a *summum bonum* or common medium in which all such conflicts may be dissolved.

In the nature of the case, however, the reasons offered for resolving a conflict among principles in a pluralistic system will not themselves appeal to some further normative principle.

For if a further normative principle could be used to rank or select among competing principles, the system would to that extent be monistic rather than pluralistic.

Instead, the judgments by which conflicts are decided will be in some way "non-principled:" that is, not themselves supported by a principle or rule. If so, then several critical questions arise that challenge the adequacy of principle-driven reasoning. What could be the nature of these judgments? How could a non-principled judgment be reasoned, when ordinary reasoning appeals to rules? If non-principled judgments are essential features of moral reflection, what role is being served by principles? Is it principled or non-principled judgments that are supplying the justification for particular positions in medical ethics? And if it is both, how are they connected to one another?

The problems posed by conflicting principles will be discussed in the next chapter, where I address attempts to meet this challenge.

Principles Leave out Important Features of Morality

Another sort of objection to the use of principles does not find them inadequate across the board for the justification of particular positions. Rather, the charge is that principles are not able to do justice to the entire range of the moral judgments we make. This is most often argued to be true of the virtues. Judgments about the moral character of individuals form a significant part of our ethical repertoire, but a number of people have wanted to claim that the attribution of a virtue like "honesty" to a person is not reducible to the claim that she follows a rule about truth-telling.

Further discussion of this criticism will be found in the later chapter on virtue theories.

Principles Are not Epistemically Basic

Next one might argue that many of the particular judgments principles are alleged to support are epistemically more secure and more basic than the principles themselves.[3] This is shown by the fact that alleged principles are often most effectively criticized by showing how they imply an unacceptable moral conclusion. A stock criticism of utilitarianism, for instance, is that given the right set of circumstances, the principle of utility could justify the punishment of an innocent person in order to prevent mob violence.[4] If proper moral reasoning could proceed only by appeals to principles, this would be an improper method of criticism. It would take our moral intuition about the particular situation to be a secure ethical datum, which at least in the context does not require any further argument.

The recognition that judgments about cases are often more secure than convictions about principles leads in two possible directions. One may take this to justify adding appeals to cases to one's repertoire of methods, as a supplement to appeal to principle, rather than a replacement for it. This produces a coherence model of moral justification, in which implication moves in two directions: from principles to cases, and from cases to principles. Coherence models invite questions about how the two modes of inference work together, and in particular how to judge the import of a particular case for the system of principles surrounding it. We'll look into these further in the next chapter.

The other direction is less equivocal about the priority of case judgments, since it sees principles providing at best a derivative mode of justification. Reasoning about cases must proceed from cases, because this is where the greater ethical certainty is found. This is casuistry, which I'll be discussing in a later chapter.

At the extreme end of this line of thought one sometimes finds a cynicism about the likelihood that appeal to moral principle will offer any moral insight. Any principle that carries disconcerting implications for our particular moral convictions will necessarily be suspect. On the flip side, any principle that carries with it *no* disconcerting implications for our particular moral convictions is nothing but a reflection of those convictions. As such, it could add no weight to our confidence in them. It would be an empty gesture, for example, to argue on behalf of our belief that adult competent patients have the right to consent or to refuse consent for medical treatment by appealing to some "deeper" principle expressing a right to self-determination. If we didn't already believe in the right to consent, we wouldn't likely believe in the more general right to self-determination that provides the alleged justification. Cheryl Noble claimed some years ago that such a closed and circular system of reasons means that applied ethicists will "inevitably arrive at conventional and tame conclusions, drawn from a preexisting range of alternatives" (Noble, 1982, p. 8).

Whether applied ethicists are always conventional and tame in their conclusions can be answered only by sampling the literature, which I will leave to the reader.

Principles Are Inherently Vague

Another criticism leveled against exclusive reliance on principles is that principles are inherently vague. A principle like "Respect autonomy," while general enough to command virtually unanimous assent (these days, at least), is not specific enough to be of much use in making moral judgments about particular choices. Determining whether respect for autonomy requires that we honor a refusal of life-saving treatment by a 14-year-old will require that we fill out the moral meaning of both "autonomy" and "respect." Unless we are doing so from within a monistic theory, the interpretation that is provided for the injunction to "respect autonomy" will not be justified by any higher or more basic principle. And the principle of respect for autonomy does not carry its own interpretation with it in the literal meaning of its words.

Another version of this problem arises for any appeal to a principle of utility (whether within a utilitarian normative theory or within a pluralistic system that includes such a principle). A principle of utility requires that I choose the alternative that will produce the greatest aggregate good. But how will I decide which alternative that is? The principle of utility itself cannot tell me which it is, for the principle merely presumes that such a judgment is possible. Even after exhaustively describing the alternative sets of consequences, I can have no principled way of supporting the value judgment that one set contains greater net good than the other unless I have both a theory of the good (which, for instance, defines "good" as pleasure and "evil" as pain) and a metric providing a common denominator by means of which goods and evils can be measured, totaled, and ranked. There is no such measure, particularly for interpersonal comparisons of utility in which different kinds of goods and evils are evaluated.[5] Of course, despite this we often do make such comparative judgments. These judgments, however, are not in any articulate way based in an argument from the principle of utility.

The point is that the application of any normative principle will require value judgments that themselves lie beyond the reach of the principle, but are essential for its interpretation. This does not imply that the principle is mistaken, only that by itself it is inadequate for the task it is set to. Perhaps indeed in some context we can all agree that we should strive to maximize the aggregate good. This agreement in principle will not be of use in helping resolve disagreements, which in all likelihood will be disagreements concerning where the maximum good is to be found.

Others have noted the necessity for interpretive judgments of this kind, among them, interestingly, Kant.

> "If understanding in general is to be viewed as the faculty of rules, judgment will be the faculty of subsuming under rules... General logic contains, and can contain, no rules for judgment... If [general logic] sought to give instructions how we are to subsume under these rules... it could only be by means of another rule. This in turn, for the very reason that it is a rule, again demands guidance from judgment. And thus it appears that... judgment is a peculiar talent which can be practiced only, and cannot be taught. It is the specific quality of mother-wit [Mütterwitz]; and its lack no school can make good."
>
> (Kant, 1963, p. 177)

Recently, Charles Larmore has used Kant's argument as the point of departure to a similar conclusion about the necessity of judgment in moral reflection and argument. Like Kant, he despairs of providing any logic of judgment: "Although we can understand what kinds of situations call for moral judgment, the kinds of tasks that moral judgment is to accomplish, and the preconditions for its acquisition, there is very little positive we can say in general about the nature of moral judgment itself" (Larmore, 1987, p. 19). Yet, he insists, if moral judgment is not thoroughly rule-governed, it is not arbitrary either: "Judgment we do not exercise blindly, but rather by responding with reasons to the particularity of a given situation" (Larmore, 1987, p. 20).

Deductivism at Work: Some Examples

I will illustrate the force of some of these criticisms by examining the work of two philosophers who bring a principle-driven approach to bear on issues in medical ethics. In both cases, I will highlight the ways in which non-principled judgments are employed to provide key interpretations of the principles ostensibly doing the work of justification.

Peter Singer

The very organization of Peter Singer's book, *Practical Ethics*, reflects the idea that the establishment of basic principles is the first task of a normative ethics. Thus, before he addresses the ethics of abortion, euthanasia, or other particular issues concerning the morality of killing or letting die, he feels compelled to provide a principled answer to the larger question "what's wrong with killing?"

In the chapter that bears this title, Singer develops arguments on behalf of several key principles, which are in turn taken to be supported by the principle of utility. First, it is specially wrong to kill a person (a being capable of having preferences about its future existence) who prefers to continue living, because it is wrong to violate the preference of any being, unless the preference is outweighed by contrary preferences (Singer, 1993, p. 94). It is also wrong to take the life of a non-person capable of pleasure and pain when doing so will reduce the total pleasure found in the world (which he calls the "total" view), or when it would shorten the pleasurable life of a being who already exists (which he calls the "prior existence" view) (Singer, 1993, pp. 103 ff.). Neither of these interpretations of the principle of utility is entirely satisfactory, Singer admits. The total view implies that there is a duty to bring as many pleasant lives into existence as is consistent with a world in which pleasant life is still possible. Such a duty seems to proscribe contraception in most circumstances. The prior existence view avoids this problem by declaring that the pleasure of possible lives is irrelevant to our utilitarian deliberations. Singer takes this to imply the correlative proposition that the pain of possible lives is also morally irrelevant. The uncomfortable consequence that would follow is that there is no duty to avoid creating lives marked by overwhelming suffering.

Following this theoretical discussion, Singer takes up the question of abortion, among other contentious issues. After disposing of some more conventional conservative and liberal arguments, he turns to a defense of his own view. The first key claim is that we should "value [the life of the fetus] on the same scale as the lives of beings with similar characteristics who are not members of our species"; species membership plays no role in any adequate account of the wrongness of killing (Singer, 1993, p. 150). Moreover, since a fetus lacks the capacity for any conscious experience before 18 weeks, Singer says, "only after that time... does [it] need protection from harm, on the same basis as sentient, but not self-conscious, non-human animals need it" (Singer, 1993, p. 165).

But what about the potential a fetus has to become a person, a self-conscious being whose preferences will be of special value? This appeal to the potentiality of the fetus is specious, he argues. Among other things, it implies that there is a duty to bring more persons into existence, and so it has the same problem as the "total" form of utilitarianism that Singer had earlier discussed. (Singer, 1993, p. 155).

Finally, Singer acknowledges that his arguments dismissing any duties to sustain the lives of fetuses imply as well that there is no intrinsic value to the life of an infant, a conclusion that collides with a deeply held conviction to the contrary. This traditional moral conviction offers no real grounds for challenging his view, Singer asserts, urging us to remember "that our present absolute protection of the lives of infants is a distinctively

Christian attitude rather than a universal ethical value" (Singer, 1993, p. 172).

Just how adequate are Singer's *principles* for supporting his views about the ethics of abortion? In answering this question, we want to pay special attention to whether and how those principles are interpreted, and whether the principles and their interpretations are warranted by Singer's theory, or instead rely upon a non-principled appeal to particular moral intuitions.

Let's first see how well the principles he defends regarding the wrongness of killing support his claim that the fetus' life is of no intrinsic value that would make it wrong to kill it. On Singer's utilitarian principles it is wrong (other things being equal) to take the life of a being capable of future pleasures or satisfactions, from either the total or the prior existence perspective. But from either of those perspectives, wouldn't the life of the fetus have some utilitarian value that would make it *prima facie* wrong to kill it?

On the total view, it would ordinarily be wrong to kill a fetus that could be expected to develop into a person leading a decent life, because that would reduce the total amount of pleasure or preference satisfaction in the world, something that is ordinarily wrong to do. This seems a straightforward application of the principle of utility, but Singer rejects this conclusion. One of his explanations is that the total view regarding the wrongfulness of killing is unacceptable because it implies not only that abortion is wrong, but also that contraception is wrong, since that too will reduce the number of happy persons in the world. But if our moral judgments are to be derived from our principles, and not vice versa, why shouldn't we accept the stern conclusion that the total view leads to? Singer doesn't provide any principled answer to this question. Rather, he assumes as a secure moral datum the intuition that there is nothing wrong with contraception, the Roman Catholic Church notwithstanding. His argument on the ethics of abortion, therefore, is not grounded simply in an appeal to higher-level principle. It relies as well on a non-principled moral commitment that is used to limit the scope of this version of the principle of utility.

Here a utilitarian like Singer might reply by making a utilitarian case in favor of contraception, by pointing out, among other things, the tremendous value that control over childbearing would have for those whose preferences are to avoid having children.[6] But such an argument could not show that the total view is wrong in its assessment of the *prima facie* value of fetal life, only that the total view (like any other form of utilitarianism) must take into account the total range of effects that an action or rule would have on utility.

Now, what about the prior existence view, which has the virtue of avoiding the embarrassing proscription of contraception? Wouldn't it also imply that the fetus is intrinsically valuable, making it wrong ordinarily to kill it? The fetus is an existing being whose future pleasures and satisfactions will be eliminated by its death.[7] In this utilitarian respect, killing a normal human fetus is no different than killing an existing person. The only difference, from the utilitarian perspective that Singer has advanced, is that when I kill a person I usually do the additional wrong of frustrating her preference for continuing to live. This may suggest a difference in the degree of wrong done, but it can't support Singer's claim that killing a fetus is morally unproblematic, while killing a person remains a great moral wrong. It can't support the claim, that is, without the importation of some additional premises that further interpret the prior existence version of the principle of utility. One might claim that the fetus does not count as "an existing being" for purposes of applying the prior existence principle. One might say that the only future utilities that matter are those belonging to beings who are now conscious, or who are now persons.[8] Or one might say that the particular preference regarding the continuation of one's life is the only utility relevant to the wrongfulness of killing. Some such additions are essential for filling out Singer's argument, but either they are violations of the principle of utility or they are incapable of being supported by it.[9] In any event, their necessity highlights the inadequacy of exclusive reliance upon the foundational principle that Singer claims as the basis for his position.

In concluding the discussion of Singer, I want to emphasize the role that non-principled convictions play in his account. We've already seen how his claim about contraception is used to limit the "total" view's application of the principle of utility. Similarly unargued convictions play critical roles elsewhere in his argument as well. Take Singer's claim about the wrongfulness of killing a person.

> "taking the life of a person will normally be worse than taking the life of some other being, since persons are highly future-oriented in their preferences. To kill a person is therefore, normally, to violate not just one, but a wide range of the most central and significant preferences a being can have."
>
> (Singer, 1993, p. 95)

This is a non sequitur unless we assume that the particular preferences had by persons normally outweigh all the other sorts of preference utilities that would be frustrated in killing another sort of creature. But why, for example, must a *preference utilitarian* conclude that it will be worse to kill a person with a short remaining life span than to kill an elephant with a long remaining life span?

In his discussion, Singer doesn't take up this challenge directly, but he does suggest an answer in a thought experiment used to illustrate a method for determining which of two lives has greater value—in his example, the life of a horse or the life of a man. One first imagines what life would be like as a horse, and then in some third state, in between the life of a horse and the life of a man, one decides which life is preferable. It is no surprise to learn that Singer would prefer the life of a man, and draws the general conclusion that the greater the degree of rationality and self-consciousness (i.e., the more like a person), the greater the value of the life (Singer, 1993, pp. 106–107). I won't critique the cogency of this method. What is notable for my purposes is that once again a critical element of the argument comes not by derivation from any principle (let alone the principle of utility) but from an undefended moral intuition.

This reliance on intuitions is all the more surprising when put alongside Singer's dismissal of the intuition that the life of an infant has intrinsic value. Of course, the acceptance of this intuition, in contrast to those he chooses to employ, would bedevil his arguments rather than support them.

So what is really the epistemic basis for Singer's positions? It's not just the principle of utility. For that principle to be applied to the complexity of the issues Singer confronts, its interpretation must be filtered through a set of already existing moral convictions or intuitions. This doesn't mean that the principle does no work in the argument. The principle requires that reasons be concerned with and answerable to the maximization of preference satisfaction. This directs our attention to a particular feature of the situation as morally salient, and it either rules out or subordinates other considerations. But by itself, the principle is too abstract and leaves open critical questions about its application. As we've seen, it doesn't tell us how preferences are to be ranked relative to one another, and it doesn't tell us which beings are to count as having preferences. These critical questions are answered by assumptions that originate outside the principle that relies on them.

H. Tristram Engelhardt

H. Tristram Engelhardt's influential book *The Foundations of Bioethics* provides further illustrations of the limits of principles for the justification of particular judgments in medical ethics. Engelhardt's objective is to establish the parameters of a "secular" bioethics, based in principles to which all persons could agree, despite the religious, cultural, and other sectarian moral convictions that otherwise deeply divide them. "To ask a secular ethical question," he says, "is to seek a ground other than force for resolving moral controversies" (Engelhardt, 1996, p. 67). In the face of irreducible sectarian moral diversity, the only such ground is agreement, or permission. This principle of permission is constitutive of secular morality, and is content-less: "It commits one to no particular concrete moral view of the good life... or content-full moral obligations... It gives no value to permission [but is only] a minimal condition in relying on what it is to resolve issues among moral strangers with moral authority: consent" (Engelhardt, 1996, p. 69).

Thus, a principle of permission, requiring free consent to actions done to or for another, is the fundamental principle of a secular bioethics. Since it is content-less, however, it can't be sufficient to generate a full morality. For that one also needs to subscribe to a principle of beneficence—a commitment to do good and avoid evil. From the secular perspective, of course, this principle too has no content. Conceptions and hierarchies of good and evil are supplied by one's particular cultural or religious tradition and commitments, which cannot themselves be justified in secular terms. At best, the secular principle of beneficence implies a duty to not be malevolent. The principle of permission is often in conflict with a content-full principle of beneficence, this conflict being the primary source of ethical problems in bioethics. Since the principle of permission is the more fundamental, it properly sets limits on the exercise of beneficence.[10] Within secular morality, it is only persons who are owed a duty of permission, since it is only beings who are self-conscious, rational, and able to think of themselves as making free choices who form the secular moral community (Engelhardt, 1996, p. 139).

What implications for specific questions in medical ethics can Engelhardt legitimately draw from this laconic pair of principles alone? None, for two reasons: the unavoidable need to rely on substantive claims about good and evil, and the emptiness of the principle of permission.

Substantive Claims about Good and Evil

First, for any given issue, in order to claim that the principle of permission applies, he must argue or assume that the principle of non-malevolence does not apply. But in order to make that judgment, one must first be able to determine that the act in question is not an evil one, for someone who wills an evil act is by definition malevolent, and such a choice is then not protected by the principle of permission. And to presume that the act is not evil, I have to rely upon substantive conceptions of good and evil, openly or by stealth.

Take as examples his positions on abortion and infanticide. According to Engelhardt, secular morality can justify the claim that parents, especially women, have the right to abort their fetus. Parents also have a right to refuse medical treatment for their seriously ill infants, and since secular morality can offer no reasons against the practice, this right extends to infanticide.

Engelhardt offers two arguments in support of these claims, but I'll discuss only one of them.[11] This argument asserts that the lives of fetuses and infants (like zygotes, embryos, and non-human animals) have no independent value. On what grounds? "The more an organism's life is characterized not just by sensations but by consciousness of objects and goals, the more one can plausibly hold that the organism's life has value for it. The more an organism can direct itself with appreciation and subtlety to certain objects and away from others, the more plausible it is that it has an inner life with some pre-reflective anticipations of values, as values are understood by self-conscious free agents" (Engelhardt, 1996, p. 143).

Fetuses and at least newborn infants lack these attributes, and so have no special value in secular morality. "It is for these reasons in general secular morality that the value of zygotes, embryos, and fetuses is to be primarily understood in terms of the values they have for actual persons." (Engelhardt, 1996, p. 143) This premise is extended as well to infants. Although Engelhardt suggests (inexplicably, given his secular premises!) that infants perhaps should be granted a special intermediate moral standing as "persons for social consideration," even this is to be grounded in utilitarian consideration of the interests of persons proper (Engelhardt, 1996, pp. 146–151).

This is an argument at odds with the foundations of his secular morality. It employs the assumptions that the lives of *persons* have a special value, and that the value of other lives is properly benchmarked by reference to persons. This is a content-full assertion about what is good. It can't be derived from the principle of beneficence, which is content-less. And it can't be derived from the principle of permission, which is a principle of forbearance only that does not attach any positive value to freedom or to those things freely chosen: "Respect of freedom as the necessary condition for the very possibility of mutual respect... is not dependent on any particular value or ranking of goods" (Engelhardt, 1996, p. 106).

These principles can say nothing at all about the value of the lives of fetuses or infants, because they can't by themselves say anything at all about the value of the lives of persons or the things persons prefer. At most, they can forbid the proscription of abortion or infanticide, since *prima facie* this would violate the principle of permission. But they can't support any refinement or limitation on this freedom. In particular, they can't support limiting the withdrawal of treatment or infanticide to those cases in which the infant is seriously ill or faces a bleak future. In this way, they become largely irrelevant to secular bioethics as it is practiced in the United States. At some level Engelhardt must recognize this, because in his book he includes discussion of the factors, including prognosis and quality of life, usually believed to be ethically relevant to decisions to limit care because they determine whether the life in question could be a good one.

This need to employ some substantive conceptions of the good and of the value of human life, despite his theoretical strictures, leads to some stark incongruities. On the one hand, for example, he claims that "the duty to preserve the life of a newborn is generally defeated as the chance for success diminishes, as the quality or quantity of life for the newborn decreases, and as the costs of securing that quality of life increase" (Engelhardt, 1996, p. 265). Confining ourselves to his secular principles, what duty could he be referring to, since he says (on the other hand) that "General secular morality, which draws its authority and substance from the permission or concurrence of moral agents, cannot give standing to the wrongness of any intentions [regarding taking the lives of infants] save those of direct malevolence" (Engelhardt, 1996, p. 269).

The "duty" to preserve infant life in the circumstances Engelhardt describes can only be grounded by an implicit assumption that a parent who painlessly kills his healthy infant is acting malevolently. It is only after the importation of some such content-full conception of good and evil that Engelhardt has something substantive to say about the ethics of treatment limitations or infanticide.

There is a smuggled conception of the good lying behind his position on abortion as well, because he assumes that the only morally relevant interests are those of the parents. In particular, it is irrelevant whether "others would gladly adopt the child [the fetus] would become" (Engelhardt, 1996, p. 256). Even though this interest in adoption is an interest of persons who would normally therein acquire some moral standing, it is apparently not malevolent for parents to act without any regard for this interest. This cannot be a claim based on a content-less secular morality.

Emptiness of the Principle of Permission

The second problem plaguing Engelhardt's theory is the vague emptiness of the principle of permission itself. Remember that in Engelhardt's theoretical account, this principle arises from the renunciation of force, suggesting that we violate the principle any time we act against the resistance or objection of another. Engelhardt thinks that the principle of permission thus has a determinacy of meaning that the principle of beneficence lacks: "One can know when one is violating the morality of mutual respect, even when one cannot know, because of its lack of content, whether one is violating the principle of beneficence" (Engelhardt, 1996, p. 124). This is why the principle of permission has priority over the principle of beneficence.

But the principle of permission will be unambiguous only if it refers to nothing beyond mere consent or lack of opposition. At one point, Engelhardt himself makes this interpretation, when he says that "the right not to be treated without one's consent gains applicability at once from the wishes of the possible patient. It is enough for that individual to refuse in order to indicate that the authority of the physician does not extend to that patient" (Engelhardt, 1996, p. 127).

These claims are obviously false, since there are many beings (human and non-human) that have the capacity to refuse or oppose, but that aren't brought under the protection of the principle of permission, not even by Engelhardt. Young children, the insane, and the mentally retarded are cases in point. When medical treatment or other intervention is judged to be in their interests, and they are determined not to have the capacity for self-determination, they are granted no right to refuse. To justify this, the principle of permission has to be supplemented with an account that explains whose refusal or opposition matters. Engelhardt thinks he's done this by arguing for the moral primacy of "persons," abstractly understood (Engelhardt, 1996, pp. 135 ff.). It is persons who have the protection of the principle of permission, then. But the qualities that Engelhardt ascribes to persons all come in degrees. Surely, the principle of permission is granted not only to exemplars of personhood (of which there are none in fact), but to beings occupying a vast territory in which many degrees and combinations of these qualities are represented.

Neither the principle of permission nor any abstract conception of personhood can tell me in any particular case whether *this* individual is a person owed the principle of permission. Is a depressed and mildly demented lady refusing surgery for a gangrenous leg a "person" with a right to refuse? Answering the question demands an interpretation of the meaning of the concept of person as that is relevant to a right to refuse treatment (because clearly she remains a "person" in a number of other ways). Making that interpretation—determining that she is "competent" to refuse—involves the use of a moral judgment that is not contained within the literal language of either the abstract conception or the stated principle. Engelhardt's method can tell me that exemplary persons have a right to refuse, but that doesn't address the issues at stake in most concrete ethical problems. One is not surprised, then, when a glance at the index reveals that "competence" is a term often employed, but little explained.

The virtual irrelevancy of Engelhardt's brand of theorizing is illustrated by his commentary on "Dax's Case," a case well known within medical ethics.[12] "Dax" (then Donald) Cowart had been severely burned in a natural gas explosion that left him blind, partially deaf, and disfigured. He persistently demanded that treatment for his burn-related infections be stopped, even though his life could most certainly be saved if his treatment continued. Engelhardt frames the moral question as "once the patient is reasonably able to choose, should one respect a patient's request to refuse life-saving therapy even if one has good reason to believe that later the patient might change his mind?" (Engelhardt, 1975, p. 52). Having cast the issue into the only form suitable to his secular theory, Engelhardt easily derives the obvious answer: "when the patient who is able to give free consent does not, the moral issue is over" (Engelhardt, 1975, p. 53).

A tidy conclusion that is beside the point. The central issues that the case raises concern what it means "to be able to give free consent" or be "reasonably able to choose," and how particular aspects of Dax's history, psychology, and behavior might bear on our understanding of those ideas and the ethics of honoring his refusal. Engelhardt's answer assumes that these judgments are all morally unproblematic, as his theory must assume in order to begin operation at all. This disconnection from the moral life of the actual situation is epitomized by the fact that in his commentary, Engelhardt brings into play not a single particular feature of the circumstances; he doesn't even use Dax's name.[13] The inability of Engelhardt's theory to engage particular moral problems remains even after twenty years. One won't find any but the sketchiest of case discussions in *The Foundations of Bioethics*.

Summary

Singer's and Engelhardt's principle-driven approaches illustrate how significant the problem of interpretation will be for any method that bases ethical reasoning in appeals to abstract, general principles. To the extent that the necessary interpretations are founded in unargued moral judgments or intuitions, they raise the possibility that at its core, such ostensibly principle-based reasoning is sham, merely a cover for dependence upon an existing common morality. This may be a particular danger for systems like Singer's and Engelhardt's. With only one or two foundational principles, there aren't enough resources to evaluate and justify the variety of moral judgments that must be employed to interpret the core principles.

One of the attractions of a more pluralistic set of principles is to remedy this problem with a richer range of principled resources. But that creates its own set of problems, which we will discuss in the next chapter.

Notes

1. Utilitarians come in different flavors, of course. They may apply the principle of utility to a system of rules, or to specific acts. And they differ in the nature of the "good" they seek to maximize.

2. See Kekes' (1993) discussion of the differences between monistic and pluralistic systems.

3. One variety of this view is held by Edmund Pincoffs, who argues that there are a number of moral "truisms" (e.g., cruelty is wrong) that are more certain than any more general or theoretical justification that might be given for them (Pincoffs, 1986, Ch. 4).

4. See Rachels' (1993) discussion of counterexamples to consequentialism, p. 105 ff.

5. See Kekes' (1993) discussion.

6. Thanks to Martin Benjamin for reminding me of this tactic.

7. Note that since this argument does not refer to the *aggregate* utility, it avoids Singer's principal objection to appeals to the potentiality of the fetus.

8. This is the upshot of a tortuous defense of the idea that the prior existence interpretation should be applied only to self-conscious beings, because it is only in the case of non-self conscious-beings that the loss of value caused by the death of an existing being can be compensated for by the creation of a new being bearing new pleasures and satisfactions. Self-conscious beings are thus not "replaceable" in the way that other creatures are who are mere receptacles of pleasures or satisfactions. Singer says, "with non-self -onscious life, birth and death cancel each other out; whereas with self-conscious beings the fact that once self-conscious one may desire to continue living means that death inflicts a loss for which the birth of another is insufficient compensation" (Singer, 1993, pp. 126–127).

Well, of course it is no compensation for *me*, the one who dies, if as a result another being with equal or greater capacities for satisfaction is created. But it *is* a compensation for the loss to the aggregate utility that my death otherwise represents. In this respect, persons and their preference utilities are just as replaceable as non-persons, and the killing of persons or non-persons is wrong for, or justifiable for, exactly the same kinds of utilitarian reasons. But see Singer's attempt to respond to a similar objection by H. L. A. Hart (Singer, 1993, pp. 127 ff.).

9. A principle of utility contains no mention of the entities to which it is to apply, and a utilitarian who gives no thought to future consequences for the good is no utilitarian.

10. Engelhardt's arguments regarding these principles are neatly summarized toward the end of Chapter 3 (Engelhardt, 1996, pp. 122–124).

11. The other concerns who it is who has rights over the lives of fetuses (and infants). Here Engelhardt employs a conception of property: because "the parents, and especially the woman, have produced the fetus... they have a secular moral right to abort the fetus" (Engelhardt, 1996, p. 256). This obviously relies upon a value-laden Lockean conception of property not derivable from the principles of permission or beneficence.

12. See the collection of essays on Dax's case by Lonnie D. Kliever (1989). Engelhardt's essay in the collection, like his 1975 commentary, still insists on discussing the case as if it were merely an exemplar of an

abstract conflict between the duty of permission and the duty of beneficence.

13. Thanks to Susan Brown Trinidad for pointing this out to me.

Bibliography

Brink, David O. 1989. *Moral Realism and the Foundations of Ethics.* New York: Cambridge University Press.

Caplan, Arthur L. 1980. "Ethical Engineers Need Not Apply: The State of Applied Ethics Today." *Science, Technology and Human Values* 6, Fall 24–32.

Chuck, C. "Human Cloning Responses." Http://207.217.52.45/cloning.htm. Last updated 6/19/97.

Crisp, Roger. 2000. "Particularizing Particularism." In Hooker, Brad and Margaret Little. *Moral Particularism.* New York: Oxford, pp. 23–47.

Dancy, Jonathan. 1993. *Moral Reasons.* Oxford: Blackwell.

Engelhardt, H. Tristram. 1975. "A Demand to Die" (Commentary). *Hastings Center Report*, June 52–53.

Engelhardt, H. Tristram. 1996. *The Foundations of Bioethics*, 2nd ed. New York: Oxford University Press.

Frankena, William K. 1973. *Ethics*, 2nd ed. Englewood Cliffs, NJ: Prentice-Hall.

Hare, R. M. 1963. *Freedom and Reason.* London: Oxford University Press.

Hare, R. M. 1981. *Moral Thinking.* New York: Oxford University Press.

Hare, R. M. 1992. "Universalizability." In Lawrence C. and Charlotte B. Becker, eds. *Encyclopedia of Ethics.* New York: Garland Publishing.

Herman, Barbara. 1993. "The Practice of Moral Judgment." In Barbara Herman. *The Practice of Moral Judgment.* Cambridge: Harvard University Press, pp. 73–93.

Hooker, Brad and Margaret Little. 2000. *Moral Particularism.* New York: Oxford.

Kant, Immanuel. 1963. *Critique of Pure Reason.* Trans. Norman Kemp Smith. New York: St. Martin's Press.

Kekes, John. 1993. *The Morality of Pluralism.* Princeton, NJ: Princeton University Press.

Kliever, Lonnie D. 1989. *Dax's Case: Essays in Medical Ethics and Human Meaning*. Dallas: Southern Methodist University Press.

Larmore, Charles E. 1987. *Patterns of Moral Complexity*. New York: Cambridge University Press.

Noble, Cheryl N. 1982. "Ethics and Experts." *Hastings Center Report*, June 7–9.

Rachels, James. 1975. "Active and Passive Euthanasia." *New England Journal of Medicine* 292 (2): 78–80.

Rachels, James. 1993. *The Elements of Moral Philosophy*, 2nd ed. New York: McGraw-Hill.

Pincoffs, Edmund L. 1986. *Quandaries and Virtues: Against Reductivism in Ethics*. Lawrence, KS: University Press of Kansas.

Ross, W. D. 1939. *The Foundations of Ethics*. Oxford: Oxford University Press.

Singer, Peter. 1993. *Practical Ethics*, 2nd ed. London: Cambridge University Press.

Tomlinson, Thomas. 1980. *The Use of Principles in Moral Reasoning*. E. Lansing: Michigan State University (unpublished dissertation).

Toulmin, Stephen. 1970. *Reason in Ethics*. London: Cambridge University Press.

Chapter 3

Putting Principles in Context

Balancing, Specification, and Reflective Equilibrium

Principles of Biomedical Ethics, by Tom Beauchamp and James F. Childress, has for many critics exemplified the worst sins of principlism. From its first edition, the authors have argued for the importance and usefulness of general principles for justifying ethical judgments about policies and cases in medical ethics. The organization of their book reflects this conviction, dividing discussion of particular ethical problems under the rubrics of the key ethical principles that the authors believe should govern our moral judgments: principles of autonomy, nonmaleficence, beneficence, and justice.

It was always a caricature of their views to label them simple deductivists, who see justification as nothing but subsumption of cases under rules.[1] At the very least, they have from the first edition insisted on the necessity of making judgments about the proper *balance* to be struck between competing ethical commitments when they are in conflict. Since Beauchamp and Childress disavow appeal to any overarching framework from which such a balancing judgment could be derived, particular moral judgments could never for them be simple deductions from any single moral principle.

In the latest (now the sixth) edition of their book, the authors provide an expanded and more nuanced account of their theory and method, which is intended both to correct misinterpretations of their position and to address real gaps left open in their previous treatments.

As they characterize it, their theory starts with the "common morality" shared by members of society, and constructs principles and rules from considered judgments, seeking coherence through a process of reflective equilibrium. Developing this coherence will require both that principles be "specified" in the manner described by Richardson (2000) (and discussed below), and that judgments be made how best to prioritize or balance competing moral principles. (See Beauchamp and Childress, 2009, Ch. 10, esp. pp. 381–388.)

Each of the key elements of this account—reliance on the "common morality," specification, balancing, and coherence—is intended to respond to several of the criticisms leveled against principle-based methods described in the last chapter.

Briefly, Beauchamp and Childress describe their approach as follows. We start with the variety of basic norms found within our common morality. This consists of the principles, rules, virtues, rights and obligations, and particular judgments about which we can all agree. This common morality provides a starting point for our deliberation. Since the elements of this common morality are already agreed upon, there is no need to develop some further moral theory by which they are further justified. Key elements of the common morality most relevant to health care form the framework of their book. We can all agree that we should respect the values embraced by individuals and the freely made choices that flow from them; that we—and particularly physicians— should strive to help, and not hurt, others, particularly those for whom we have special responsibilities; and that we should treat fairly all those whose interests are affected by our actions. But the common morality is by itself not enough to grapple with the complexity of moral questions found in medicine, or even in everyday life. To begin with, the values and principles found in it are often very generally stated. As we saw in the last chapter, these need to be interpreted in order to establish their relevance and import for particular situations. In addition, few if any principles make categorical, absolute demands on us. Moral rules often admit of exception. Take the maxim, "Do not deceive." While cautioning us against lying, it doesn't yet explicate what is to count as "deception;" that concept may require an understanding of the circumstances under which, and the persons to whom, the truth is owed. Beauchamp and Childress offer as an example the results of a survey of physicians' willingness to misrepresent a patient's condition in order to secure insurance coverage for a screening mammography. Seventy percent were willing to document "rule out cancer" as a indication for the test, while 85% of those physicians insisted that this was not "deception" of the insurance company (Beauchamp and Childress, 2009, p. 18). These physicians weren't rejecting the common morality's injunction against deception. They were specifying it, to use the terminology coined by Richardson, and adopted by Beauchamp and Childress. The process of specification, they maintain, provides a means for explicating and justifying the application of general norms.

But specification is not enough, because it cannot eliminate the possibility of conflicting norms, even specified norms. Notoriously, for example, clinical situations arise that pose conflicts between obligations to respect autonomy, and obligations to protect patients from harm. Those situations will require a judgment about which of the competing norms should take precedence under the circumstances. These "balancing" judgments,

Beauchamp and Childress argue, are an essential complement to specification:

> "Principles, rules, and rights require *balancing* no less than *specification*. We need both methods because each addresses a dimension of moral principles and rules: *range and scope*, in the case of specification, and *weight or strength*, in the case of balancing."
> (Beauchamp and Childress, 2001, p. 18; cf. 2009, pp. 19–20)

Although they admit that balancing requires judgment, not just the application of further specified principles or rules, they claim that the use of intuition can be kept to a minimum, so that balancing judgments are themselves subject to reasoned justification.

Ultimately, the justification for both specifications and balancing judgments is rooted in their coherence within a larger framework of factual beliefs and moral commitments. Justification does not proceed only from the top down, as inference from general principles to specific cases, but from the bottom up as well. All elements of the system are open for possible revision, and are tested against one another, toward the goal of achieving as coherent a set of beliefs as is reasonably possible.

This combination offers a flexibility and richness of resources that preserves a key role for principled justification, while ameliorating, if not eliminating, the problems outlined in the previous chapter. The reliance on the common morality avoids the need to pin hopes on any single normative theory, while allowing a wide variety of moral considerations in addition to principles and rules. The necessity for interpretation and balancing of principles is acknowledged, but methods for doing so will be offered that minimize reliance on unreasoned moral intuition. A coherence model of justification permits the use of forms of argument other than inference from principles or rules, and allows for the critical evaluation of any element of the system of beliefs, saving us from uncritical acceptance of whatever the conventional morality dictates.

Despite these strengths, Beauchamp and Childress are cautious about claiming too much for their method. They deny that it can resolve all moral controversy, provide a fully articulate justification in all cases, or avoid all reliance on judgment and intuition. In what follows, we will get a clearer understanding of the nature and significance of these remaining limitations on principled justification.

Balancing Principles in Beauchamp and Childress

Let's start with balancing. The metaphor of balancing responds to those who argue that ethical justification that appeals to principles is bound to fail because of the inevitable conflicts arising among competing principles in a pluralistic system. If those conflicts cannot be adjudicated by appeal to some higher-level principle or rule, then any judgment about which norm has priority would appear to be intuitive and unreasoned—at the very least, not a judgment warranted by principle-based reasons.

Beauchamp and Childress have in the past admitted that in making balancing judgments, "some intuitive and subjective weightings are unavoidable, just as they are everywhere in life when we must balance competing goods" (Beauchamp and Childress, 1994, p. 36). At the same time, however, they still insist that "Justified acts of balancing can be supported by good reasons" (Beauchamp and Childress, 2009, p. 20). Since "reasons" are appeals to considerations that are intersubjectively verifiable (and in that sense "objective"), a central question will be the extent to which we can bring the intuitive and subjective to a minimum in giving reasons for balancing judgments.

As an illustration of the sort of "good reasons" they have in mind, the authors describe the situation of a physician faced with a choice between returning home to take her son on a promised trip to the library, or staying at the hospital to attend to a life-or-death emergency. Clearly, there are good reasons she should stay at the hospital. "A life hangs in the balance and she alone may have the knowledge to deal adequately with the circumstances. Canceling her evening with her son, distressing as it is, could be justified by this good and sufficient reason for doing what she does" (Beauchamp and Childress, 2009, p. 20).

The illustration, however, confuses having provided a good and sufficient reason for breaking the promise to her son, with having provided a reason of any kind for the claim that the obligation to save the patient's life is weightier than the obligation to keep the promise. The example relies upon the *assertion* of a balancing judgment—that it is more imperative to remain at the hospital than to keep her promise to her son—for which no *reasons* are offered. The judgment is taken as a given of commonsense morality that has no need for justification. Anyone who demanded that further reasons be given would rightly be thought a moral nincompoop.

In cases like this one, which arouse no significant disagreement about the proper balance between contending obligations, the failure to give reasons justifying that balance will be unproblematic outside the philosophy seminar. But in other sorts of cases, the moral controversy will center around differing judgments about what the proper balance should be. In those cases, simply to assert that one of the obligations constitutes a "good and sufficient reason" for overriding the other begs the question by failing to give any reason on behalf of the balancing judgment that has been made. Balancing would not then be a mode or method of justification; it would instead mark the end of reasoned justification as a tool of moral reflection.

In fact, Beauchamp and Childress themselves don't give reasons justifying the balancing judgments they make in support of their positions on particular issues. They simply assert them. This can be illustrated by the various views they espouse on issues involving potential conflicts between respect for autonomy and duties of nonmaleficence or beneficence. How does one decide what to do with such conflicts? Being moral pluralists, Beauchamp and Childress recognize no *a priori* ranking among these opposing obligations, and so the proper balance will depend on the circumstances, rather than be determined by any general rule. They acknowledge, for example, that "Respect for autonomy has only *prima facie* standing, and competing moral considerations sometimes can override this principle . . . The principle of respect for autonomy does not by itself determine what a person ought to be free to know or do or what counts as a valid justification for constraining autonomy" (Beauchamp and Childress, 2009, p. 105).

Since respect for autonomy is only a *prima facie* duty, how do Beauchamp and Childress decide when it is or is not properly overridden by weightier obligations?

Take one of their examples of justified strong paternalism. A patient has had a myelogram that shows some inconclusive evidence of a serious spinal cord condition. Confirmation will require further testing. "When the patient asks about the test results, the physician decides on grounds of beneficence to withhold potentially negative information, knowing that, on disclosure, the patient will be distressed and anxious."[2] Is this balancing judgment warranted? Again, Beauchamp and Childress provide a one-sentence answer. "This physician's act of temporary nondisclosure is morally justified, although beneficence has (temporarily) received priority over respect for autonomy" (Beauchamp and Childress, 2009, p. 215) No further reasons are offered to justify this claim. It is simply the deliverance of a moral intuition, not backed by any reasons.[3]

Another illustration is their 2001 discussion of the case of Larry McAfee, which is offered as an example of a justified assisted suicide. McAfee was ventilator-dependent and quadriplegic as a result of an automobile accident. At the time described in the example, McAfee wanted to be disconnected from his ventilator, and wanted to have access to the sedatives that would make it possible for him to carry out his intention to die by this means.[4] Beauchamp and Childress strongly endorse the Georgia court finding "that McAfee's right to refuse treatment and disconnect himself outweighed the state's interest in the preservation of life and in preventing suicide" (Beauchamp and Childress, 2001, p. 150).

They offered no accounting for this balancing judgment. One would seem to be called for, in light of their discussion of "justified paternalism" in the chapter that follows. There they assert that "in general, as the risk to a patient's welfare increases or the likelihood of an irreversible harm increases, the likelihood of a justified paternalistic intervention correspondingly increases." They acknowledge, moreover, that "some cases of justified hard paternalism may cross the line of minimal infringement (of autonomy)" (Beauchamp and Childress, 2009, p. 216). Given that what's at stake is McAfee's life and the possibilities for future achievements and satisfactions that it may hold, why can't a decision not to honor his demand to discontinue the ventilator or his demand for sedatives be justified on paternalistic grounds?

The recourse to "balancing" does not answer this question with a set of reasons providing a justification. It answers it by the assertion of what is taken to be obvious to moral common sense. As the controversy about a case like McAfee demonstrates, however, this will gain us nothing when we are in conversation with those whose moral common sense delivers a different intuition about where the proper balance lies.

My discussion of Beauchamp and Childress' treatment of balancing has so far left out a prominent element in their account: "To allay concerns that the model of balancing is too intuitive or too open-ended and lacking in a commitment to firm principles and rigorous reasoning, we here list six minimal conditions that must be met to justify infringing one prima facie norm to adhere to another." They then list those conditions:

"1. Good reasons can be offered to act on the overriding norm rather than on the infringed norm.

2. The moral objective justifying the infringement has a realistic prospect of achievement.

3. No morally preferable alternative actions are available.

4. The lowest level of infringement, commensurate with achieving the primary goal of the action, has been selected.

5. Any negative effects of the infringement have been minimized.

6. All affected parties have been treated impartially.

(Beauchamp and Childress, 2009, p. 23)

We can begin by setting aside the first and last criteria. The first can't count as a *reason for* a balancing judgment. If the "good reasons" it refers to include the balancing judgments Beauchamp and Childress believe are in fact essential for good ethical reasoning, then it is hard to see how this first criterion for a good balancing judgment would avoid begging the question. The last is a gratuitous addition. Of course, all parties should be treated "impartially." Since Beauchamp and Childress provide no further explanation of this last condition, I'll not trouble with it further myself.

The remaining criteria are not criteria for evaluating a balancing judgment. Rather, they are criteria for comparing courses of action with respect to selecting the one that entails the least infringement of all the norms at stake, *without regard to which norm is the weightier*. If the second condition is not met, for example, it follows that the alternative of not infringing the norm is the course of action that results in less infringement of the norms I value, and so should be preferred. It would make no sense to infringe norm A in order to achieve norm B when I'm not likely even to achieve norm B. If I don't infringe norm A, at least one of my norms is achieved, rather than neither of them. To make this evaluation, I don't have to make any judgment about which norm would be the more important if in fact I could achieve the one by sacrificing the other. Similarly for the third, fourth, and fifth conditions. If they are not met, then there is an alternative course of action that offers less of an infringement of norms, because the conflict between the norms in question either disappears or is reduced.

When all of the criteria are satisfied, they establish that there is an irreducible conflict between norms that *only then* will require a judgment about which norm should be overriding. At that point, however, the criteria are of no further use in warranting the balancing judgment that must follow. In the sixth edition, Beauchamp and Childress suggest that these are necessary conditions ("must be met") for a justified balancing judgment. They are right. Until these conditions are met, no balancing judgment is called for; but the conditions don't justify the balancing judgment that follows.

Take as an example Beauchamp and Childress' evaluation of policies for mandatory premarital screening for HIV infection, required for a while in several states, and discussed by them in some detail in the fourth edition of their book. In their argument against such policies, they pointed out that screening of this population identifies only a few cases that more efficient voluntary means couldn't identify; that there's no evidence that such policies prevent additional HIV infection or illness; and that spouses and future offspring can be better protected by counseling and voluntary testing (Beauchamp and Childress, 1994, pp. 414–415). These are arguments that mandatory testing is unjustified because there are morally better alternatives that infringe *neither* duties of respect for autonomy *nor* duties of beneficence or nonmaleficence. They are not arguments that decide what we should do in the event there were no such alternatives—that is, in the event we really had to prioritize between competing moral objectives.

I am not denying that these criteria are useful in the moral evaluation of options. As necessary conditions for any defensible claim about prioritizing norms, they are a tool for criticizing and rejecting claims or policies. They would, for example, provide a framework for responding to someone who argued on behalf of mandatory testing by asserting that rights to autonomy should yield to concerns to protect public health. This assertion, even if taken to be true as a matter of principle, is irrelevant if in fact these norms are not in conflict. We may also employ the framework provided by these criteria more positively, to aid in the refinement of approaches that achieve a compromise between otherwise conflicting moral perspectives.

These criteria, and forms of critical moral reasoning they support, are made possible by the adoption of *prima facie* principles as one basis for moral reflection. To the extent that we see ourselves bound by multiple general values or commitments, we are motivated to look for ways in which all or most of those commitments can be honored—to minimize our moral losses. We don't have to believe in the possibility of reasoned balancing judgments to employ this critical strategy, only in the pull of principles.

More Balancing: Clouser and Gert

The late K. Danner Clouser and Bernard Gert were persistent critics of Beauchamp and Childress' principle-based view. Indeed, they coined the pejorative use of the term "principlism." The main thrust of their critique is that the so-called principles are little more than "chapter headings." They are terms that loosely group together a variety of moral features. "A principle [as used by Beauchamp and Childress] functions mainly as a check list of considerations," which are not ordered by any larger theory. As a result, such "principles" can provide no "specific direction for action" (Clouser and Gert, 1990, p. 222). For example, they complain that "the" principle of beneficence in Beauchamp and Childress is merely "a label for a general concern with consequences" of many different sorts: some are concerned with conferring benefit; others with preventing harm; some are limited by special role duties; others are more generally binding (Clouser and Gert, 1990, p. 226). Since the weight and scope of these disparate considerations are so indeterminate, "the" principle of beneficence does not provide a clear directive for action in the same way as, say, the principle of utility does.

The alternative they advocate is Gert's system of moral rules, which he has developed over a number of years. On Gert's view, "a justified moral system is one that all impartial rational persons, using only those beliefs that are shared by all rational persons, would advocate adopting as a public system that applies to all rational persons" (Gert, 1988, pp. 282–283).[5] Furthermore, there is a limited set of ten specific moral rules that he argues are binding on all rational persons. These include such injunctions as "Don't kill," "Don't cause pain," "Don't deceive," and "Obey the law."

Since these rules enjoin particular actions, they provide guidance that the more nebulous moral principles cannot. They are not, however, absolute. As Gert explains, "Everyone is always to obey the rule except when an impartial rational person can advocate that violating it be publically allowed" (Gert, 1988, p. 284).

How do we determine that this condition is satisfied? We determine whether "publically allowing [a] violation would result in more evil being suffered than not publically allowing it" (Gert, 1988, p. 285). If it would result in more evil, then no rational person could advocate the violation of the rule. If it would result in more good, or less evil, then all rational persons would advocate the violation. And if rational persons disagree whether the violation would result in more evil than good, then at least some rational persons will advocate the violation, and the condition will at least weakly be satisfied.

Despite Clouser's and Gert's claims for it, it is hard to see how this system of moral rules offers any advantages over Beauchamp and Childress' pluralistic set of principles. In particular, like Beauchamp and Childress, Gert relies on balancing judgments in evaluating whether a violation of a moral rule is justified.[6]

Take his discussion of the justification of paternalistic deception. There he uses the example of a woman who has just been diagnosed by her doctor to have inoperable cancer. She is about to begin a long-awaited vacation. She asks her doctor what is wrong. Should the doctor tell her the blunt truth, or temporize by saying that he is not yet sure, but will have more information when she returns in two weeks?

According to Gert, the second option "is the wrong answer. It is wrong because no rational impartial person would publically allow one person to deceive another in order to prevent unpleasant feelings when the person to be deceived has a rational desire to know the truth. . . It amounts to publically allowing deception in order to impose one's own ranking of evils on others who have an alternative rational ranking." No rational person could advocate this because "publically allowing this kind of violation would have far worse consequences on any rational ranking than not publically allowing it" (Gert, 1988, p. 289).

Let's start by assuming that Gert means to be speaking about the balance of consequences of a violation of the moral rule against deception in this *specific* sort of instance—a doctor delays revealing the truth about a patient's condition in order to avoid or ameliorate distress. Note that not all rational impartial persons appear to agree with Gert's assessment of that balance. First, and as he acknowledges, physicians have at least traditionally taken a different view of the matter, favoring the prevention of excessive or undue distress over scrupulously blunt disclosure of the whole truth and nothing but.[7] Nothing in Gert's discussions of "impartiality" implies that physicians (or patients) are *ipso facto* partial in their judgment in this regard simply because each of them occupies a position that may give them a particular point of view.[8] Second, recall that Beauchamp and Childress, in a similar case discussed earlier involving a patient who wanted to receive the results of a myelogram, reached quite a different conclusion regarding the balance of consequences. Gert gives no more reasons to support his balancing judgment than Beauchamp and Childress do to support theirs. Just like them, when it comes to hard cases, Gert's moral conclusion appears to rest on an intuition that's taken for granted, rather than a set of reasons.

Such an intuition may become less problematic when Gert shifts the moral focus of the question. He starts with a particular instance of medical paternalism, but ends with a question about a completely general principle allowing deception in any circumstance in which the deceiver believes that the deceived would be better off. Perhaps indeed all rational persons agree that such a global exception to the rule against deception would leave us worse off. But what's the relevance of that judgment to the case presented? The case involves a decision to deceive temporarily in order to preserve an opportunity for pleasure, while still leaving time for the patient to put her life in order once the full truth is known.[9] Because the circumstances of the case are so narrowly constrained, it is perfectly possible that one might believe an exception to the moral rule against deception would have positive consequences here, while rejecting such a judgment in the more general case. To rely upon a less controversial balancing judgment, Gert has paid the price of irrelevance.

Beauchamp and Childress, Clouser and Gert, and indeed all pluralistic systems of principles may have to rely on balancing judgments to resolve particular cases. But if balancing judgments invoke intuitions about which norms are weightier, then they mark the boundary at which principled reflection and justification have stopped. As Henry Richardson notes, this is a problem if we believe that ethical "justifications must be offered in terms of reasons that may be publicly stated." To the extent that we cannot articulate our justifications in this way, we frustrate the ability of others to build on our insights, or draw implications from them for new cases (Richardson, 2000, p. 286). Is there a way to decide conflicts between principles without resorting to a wholly intuitive balancing?

Specifying Norms

Recall from the last chapter that one key criticism of principlism points to the gap that is found between a necessarily vague general principle and the specifics of the particular cases that the principle is called upon to resolve. To establish the relevance of such principles to particular cases, the principles will need to be interpreted in a way that links them to particular sets of circumstances. How are those interpretations to be justified?

In his influential discussion, Henry Richardson helpfully points out that not all instances in which a general principle is

related to a more specific one are properly called "interpretations" of the general norm. "Interpretation" properly refers to a
case in which the original, general norm is itself modified to
make its application to a more particular set of facts clear. When
we "derive" a more specific principle from a general one, we are
not interpreting it (Richardson, 2000, pp. 288–289). We can
derive either by "deductive subsumption" or by causal reasoning.
An example of the first is to derive a *prima facie* rule against
revealing a patient's sexual problems from a more general rule
requiring confidentiality of a patient's private information.
Sexual problems are already understood to be an instance of
"private information," and once this is given, the more specific
norm follows from the general one by deduction. An example of
the second is a rule requiring that nurses not leave messages
containing medical details on an answering machine. Since one
knows that persons other than the patient may have access to
the machine, leaving such messages creates too high a likelihood
of causing a breach of the general norm of confidentiality.

"Specification" is Richardson's term for a process by which a
general norm is "interpreted," properly so called. Specification is
designed to offer a key advantage over derivation as a method of
articulating more specific rules. In his original 1990 article,[10]
Richardson notes that the demand for interpreting a general
principle often arises in circumstances where it may conflict with
other principles and norms. Resolution of the problem will
require that one or more of these ethical commitments be modified. This is a task that derivation cannot handle, since deriva-
tions concern only the implications of individual principles.

Richardson is critical of methods that ask us simply to weigh
the competing norms in a balancing judgment, since (as we've
already seen) these judgments are unreasoned and intuitive.
Instead, he argues that we should resolve the conflict by providing a more specific interpretation of one or more of the principles

at stake. He sets conditions on these specifications to ensure that the favored resolution is not achieved by a merely *ad hoc* interpretation (e.g., by appending "or" or "and" conditions that bear no relation to the original norm). In describing the advantages of this method, he notes that specification gives "us a way to articulate how a specific norm is meaningfully related back to a more abstract one," and how in turn the resolution of the concrete case is based on a commitment to the otherwise vague general norm or principle (Richardson, 1990, p. 297).

In his original article, Richardson provides several illustrative examples of specification. Examination of one of these will help in understanding and evaluating the method.

Richardson describes a case involving a decision by its parents to withhold nutrition and hydration from a seriously ill newborn, and notes that there are three principles in contention:

1. A prohibition on directly killing innocent persons
2. A duty to respect the reasonable choices of parents regarding their children
3. A duty of health care workers to benefit rather than harm the infant and its parents.

After stipulating or bracketing answers to a number of contentious side issues (e.g., whether withholding of treatment is the same sort of thing as direct killing), Richardson describes how specification could resolve the conflict.

The first step is for the deliberator to ask herself what the grounds are for the prohibition on killing. When she does so, she may conclude that it is based in a more general principle of respect for self-conscious life. Furthermore, the present circumstances lead her to appreciate how continued life might no longer be a good for the person living it. These considerations motivate her to further specify (1), so that it reads "It is generally wrong directly to kill innocent human beings who have attained self-consciousness, and generally wrong directly to kill human beings with the . . . potential to develop self-consciousness who would not be better off dead" (Richardson, 1990, p. 304). Thus specified, the initially vague principle forbidding the taking of innocent human life (1) would permit a decision to withhold food and fluids in cases in which an infant had no prospect of developing self-consciousness, or suffered so terribly that it would be better off dead.

Clearly, specification has here provided a link between a general principle and a specific ethical problem. But this is a purely formal, logical feature of the method: such a link is merely what specification asks us to construct. What is less clear is whether principles thus specified carry the force of a justification. This is especially problematic for principles in a pluralistic system.

To see the problem, start by asking how it is that a particular specification of a general norm is to be itself justified. In Richardson's example, a key step in the specification of (1) assumes that the prohibition on killing is justified by appeal to a yet more general principle (respect for persons), which can in turn be specified to refer to respect for self-conscious life. What is notable about this is the implicit assumption that behind every principle requiring specification is a more fundamental norm providing the terms in which the specification will be carried out. This assumption is warranted only to the extent that one has in hand a viable monistic normative theory (like Richardson's implicit Kantianism). By contrast, if the normative system is a pluralistic one containing a number of basic moral principles that are taken to be moral givens (like that adopted by Beauchamp and Childress), no specification of them can be justified by appeal to any more basic or general norm.

How then could a particular specification be justified in a pluralistic system? Richardson's discussion suggests one answer, but it's not a very happy one given his rejection of balancing. His specification of the prohibition on killing provides an exemption for killings done in cases where a potentially self-conscious being would be "better off dead." What justifies the inclusion of this consideration? For Richardson's deliberator, "the present practical conflict leads her to qualify the revised prohibition on killing further by reference to the principle of benefit" (Richardson, 1990, p. 304). But if the goal of the specification is to dissolve the *prima facie* conflict between these two principles, note that there is another alternative. One might elect to preserve the core prohibition on killing by specifying the principle of benefit to prohibit judgments that a person can be better off dead than alive.[11] It seems that in all cases of conflicting principles, there would be multiple routes by which the conflict could be resolved by specification. In his later article, Richardson acknowledges that "the bare idea of specification does not indicate how one ought to specify principles so as to resolve a concrete problem. . . [because] multiple alternative, incompatible resolutions might be reached by specifying" (Richardson, 2000, p. 302).

What could be the basis for a choice between such alternatives? One possibility is that the choice relies on a judgment about which principle has priority in the circumstances. If it is the principle of benefit, then it is the prohibition on killing that will be specified, and vice versa. The specification, in other words, would rest upon a balancing judgment, with all of the difficulties just discussed. If the balancing judgment were itself unproblematic, the specification it justified would be superfluous, since the priority set in the balancing judgment would alone determine what we should do in a particular case. If Richardson's deliberator believes that in the circumstances the principle of benefit should have priority, she has no need to specify the prohibition on killing to know what to do.

There is an ironic parallel here with Richardson's criticism of Gert, Culver, and Clouser's use of balancing judgments. After describing their reliance on the question whether a particular violation of a rule will result in less harm than following it, he declares that he is left with "the suspicion that what is actually happening is that [they] are noticing which moral conclusions we actually come to and then *reading off* from those judgments the assertion that we judge one harm to be greater than another. If this is the case . . . then judgments of relative harm can never provide a *way* of determining which norm overrides" (Richardson, 2000, p. 297; original italics). The claim that a particular balance of harms exists neither explains nor increases our confidence in the moral judgment that it allegedly supports.

The justification that specification offers threatens to be equally impotent when the choice between competing specifications depends upon a balancing judgment, unless one can point to some force of justification that a specification carries, but not the corresponding balancing judgment. Richardson thinks that this additional advantage is provided by the discursive explicitness of a specification. Because they are stated as principles, "specifications can be defended on the basis of reflective equilibrium: by making arguments that show how they may [or may not] be supported by their fit with what we continue to believe on due reflection" (Richardson, 2000, p. 302).

But can specification avoid intuitive balancing judgments through the use of reflective equilibrium?

Coherence and Wide Reflective Equilibrium

Both Richardson and Beauchamp and Childress agree that specification and balancing by themselves are not adequate for warranting a particular moral conclusion. As we've seen, each of these methods is indeterminate in its application, since neither has the resources to decide between *competing* specifications or balancing judgments. The additional element they look to is coherence, in the form of a "wide reflective equilibrium." Richardson proposes "a coherence standard for the rationality of specification. This standard in effect carries the Rawlsian idea of 'wide reflective equilibrium' down to the level of concrete cases." Any justifiable specification must be backed by a theory, which "makes intelligible logical connections among the norms to which one is committed that do not merely demonstrate that they are logically compatible with each other, but also explain some of them in terms of others" (Richardson, 1990, p. 300).

Beauchamp and Childress also appeal to a coherence theory to provide the standard of justification within which specifying judgments must operate: "we also need to link specification to a method of justification that allows for a reflective testing of our moral principles and other relevant moral beliefs to make them as coherent as possible" (Beauchamp and Childress, 2009, p. 19).

What is the idea behind a coherence model of justification in ethics? Basically, the model is drawn by analogy to hypothesis testing in science. There, the truth of my law-like principles and explanatory theories is not warranted by somehow comparing them with the world as it "really is." There is no way to characterize the world as it really is independently of the language of my principles and theories. What I do instead is try to construct a *system* of principles, theories, and observations that fits as many of the pieces of the puzzle together as possible. To the extent that they are interdependent, the pieces provide mutual corroboration for one another. And the more pieces of the puzzle a particular model pulls together, the more credible it is relative to its competitors. If my theory of oxidation can explain both the phenomenon of rusting (where something seems "added") and the phenomenon of burning (where something seems "lost"), then it is superior to theories that are forced to treat these as unrelated phenomena.[12]

The model of "wide reflective equilibrium," suggested by John Rawls,[13] has been most influentially elaborated by Norman Daniels (1979), who explicitly borrows coherence views of scientific justification. In Daniels' account, there are three basic elements relevant to justification in ethics. The first is a set of "considered judgments," which are the more-or-less specific moral convictions we share after some degree of moral deliberation and correction of mistaken factual beliefs. The second is a set of moral principles, which must in some measure account for the considered judgments. And the third are various background theories, which may both explain or justify general principles, and themselves be connected to and in part warranted by considered judgments.

The aim of wide reflective equilibrium is to bring all of these elements together into a coherent system. A particular considered judgment is justified insofar as it is contained within an "ordered triple" that consists of a moral principle (or set of principles) whose scope includes that considered judgment (along with others), together with a background theory or belief (or set of them) that both supports the moral principle and in turn is at least in part supported by other considered judgments that lie outside the scope of the moral principle (Daniels, 1979, p. 258).

Wide reflective equilibrium grounds the credibility of a moral judgment by explaining how that judgment is ratified by principles and theories that we accept on other grounds. In effect, coherence serves to transmit ethical credibility from one part of the system to the other.

Notice that wide reflective equilibrium offers possibilities for addressing some of the problems with principled justification noted in the previous chapter. These stem from the fact that in coherence models, justification is always inferential, but needn't be linear (using David Brink's terminology). It is always inferential, because there is no moral judgment or principle that (it assumes) must be taken as self-evident. It needn't be linear, because inference proceeds not only from the general principle to the particular case (by deduction), but also in the other direction, as when considered judgments about cases play a role in warranting claims about principles.

In the previous chapter, for example, it was noted that theorists like Singer and Engelhardt face the problem of interpretation, which in their cases was accomplished by appealing to particular moral judgments that could not themselves be justified by the basic principles being interpreted. Since there was no other available avenue for justification, they seemed the product simply of moral intuition or moral convention. On a coherence model, not only is it permissible to use particular moral judgments to modify, reject, or interpret principles; those judgments themselves do not stand above the need for justification, but can in turn be evaluated in light of their fit within the larger system. The interpretation of principles is a problem for theorists like Singer and Engelhardt because their mode of ethical justification cannot warrant the interpretations that must be made. On a coherence view, particular interpretations of principles are warranted in the same way as the principles themselves are—by their fit within the entire system of beliefs—and so there is no comparable difficulty presented by the necessity of interpretation.

Although it escapes the problem of interpretation, wide reflective equilibrium may yet stumble over other difficulties, in particular those connected to balancing judgments. To see how these arise, let's take as an example Daniels' later discussion of the claims of the elderly on health resources (Daniels, 1987).[14] The lower-level principle that Daniels wants to support is the claim that it is permissible to withhold life-prolonging treatments from the old in favor of the young. This principle fits with considered judgments about cases in which the lives of elderly people are only marginally prolonged by expensive and burdensome treatment, which Daniels illustrates with the example of his great-aunt. The principle is in turn implied by a higher-level principle of equal opportunity: that resources should be distributed to give everyone an equal opportunity for a normal range of life's opportunities.

Two background theories come into play to support this principle of equal opportunity and its interpretation. One is a theory of personal identity, which asserts that the boundaries between different persons' experiences are more ethically significant than the boundaries between different time slices of the same person's experience. This theory is in part supported by considered judgments, like ones affirming the continued moral responsibility of aged but now reformed former Nazis for the crimes of their youth.[15] The theory also explains why it is not *per se* discriminatory to allocate resources by age: the people who when older suffer the effects of fewer life-prolonging technologies are the very same people who when younger enjoyed the benefits of greater access to those technologies. At the same time, the theory makes it possible to avoid conflicts with other considered judgments within the scope of the equal opportunity principle (e.g., considered judgments against racist or sexist distributions).

The other background theory is a principle of procedural justice, which asserts that a fair process for choosing from among conflicting interests is to make sure that the decision is not "biased" from the outset in favor of one interest over others. This principle is connected to various specific considered judgments. It is also the principle embodied in the Rawlsian device of the veil of ignorance, and if those behind the veil would choose the principle of equal opportunity that Daniels advocates, then this fair procedure principle supports that intermediate moral principle, and in turn the principle permitting the use of age as a criterion for withholding life-prolonging resources from the elderly.

As the example illustrates, coherence models capture a good deal of the process by which we argue ethically. In supporting our points of view, we will often appeal both to more general considerations (either moral principles or ancillary background theories) and to the particular considered judgments taken to embody and support those principles and theories. Coherence models do not privilege some forms of moral knowledge over others, at least not in any absolute way. In so doing, they avoid the objections of those who think that particular judgments can be a more compelling source of moral knowledge than any general principle. Finally, since these models emphasize the multiple dimensions along which ethical argument can range, they capture the multi-layered and cross-disciplinary character of moral reflection.

These are considerable attractions. They should not, however, stop us from exploring the limits of this form of ethical justification. Two sets of critical questions remain. First, we want to know whether and how wide reflective equilibrium can account for the balancing judgments that seem necessary to other pluralistic systems, but that lie outside their linear modes of justification. Are balancing judgments a feature of wide reflective equilibrium? If so, can these judgments be brought within the ambit of a coherence model? Second, we will want to better understand the kind of inference used in a coherence model. Linear, deductive inference is familiar to us, and we have tools for evaluating it. But coherence models employ non-linear forms of inference. What can we say about these beyond asserting that they must exist, and how can we evaluate this kind of reasoning?

To begin answering these questions, we should ask how one reaches a justified position when there are competing coherentist arguments being deployed. Start with the simplest argument against a principle or theory: that it implies unacceptable moral conclusions. For example, we might claim that Daniels' principle implies that under conditions of scarcity it is morally permissible to withhold life-saving treatment from an otherwise healthy 75-year-old, not just Daniels' terminally ill and moribund great-aunt; and that this is morally objectionable.[16]

Such a considered judgment would throw Daniels' model into disequilibrium, requiring that somehow coherence be restored. There are always at least two routes by which equilibrium can be regained. One of these would revise the threatening considered judgment, under the warrant of the principles and background theories that imply its rejection. This is no doubt the alternative that Daniels would favor. But we should remember that one chief attraction of a coherence view is that it also explains how particular considered judgments can provide the basis for rejection of a principle or a theory. When we do, we will have to recognize that the alternative route to coherence is to keep the considered judgment, and reject one or more of the principles or theories with which it is incompatible.

Can the standard of coherence help determine which route we should take? It is hard to see how. Either alternative achieves coherence within a system of judgments, principles, and theories. In that case, deciding which way to achieve coherence will have to turn on some other consideration. That consideration, it seems to me, will be a judgment about which alternative exacts the smallest price from our felt moral sensibilities. Which is the more ethically significant—our conviction about the wrongfulness of withholding effective life-saving treatment; or our faith in the particular interpretation of the principle of equal opportunity that Daniels employs? We are back, once again, to making a balancing judgment.

This is true even if we take the measure of coherence to be something more positive than mere consistency, like the degree to which judgments, principles, and theories "mutually support" one another.[17] Someone might argue in Daniels' defense that achieving coherence by revising the considered judgment does more than achieve consistency. It ties up a larger range of moral convictions (including other considered judgments) into a more systematized whole than the alternative would.

This is unconvincing in two ways. First, it employs a normative imperative that it cannot presume to be absolute: It is better for a set of moral convictions to be more systematic rather than less. This may be a desirable goal, but is it one to be pursued at any price? If the answer is "No," then in any particular case we will have to judge whether what I will call the norm of coherence is more important than the norm to be sacrificed for its sake.

An example of this dynamic is found in some of the literatures discussing infanticide, and decisions to withhold life-sustaining treatment from newborns. Drawing on the work of Joel Feinberg, writers such as Michael Tooley and Martin Benjamin argue that in order to have a right to X, a being must be able to have an interest in X; and that in order for a being to have an interest in X, X must be the possible object of that being's desires or preferences.

This is a theory of rights and their correlative interests buttressed by appeal to a range of paradigm cases for which it can account. To use one of Tooley's examples, it can plausibly explain why "A child does not have a right to smoke" makes a sensible moral claim while "A newspaper does not have a right to be torn up" does not (Tooley, 1985, p. 98). It can provide the basis for arguing, as Feinberg does, that non-human animals have interests (and hence possible rights) of some sorts, like an interest in avoiding pain, but not of others, like a right to attend medical school. In a variety of ways such as these, it ties together a considerable chunk of our moral judgments into a more coherent system.

The principles warranted by this coherence are then employed to justify conclusions that run contrary to deeply held moral convictions. Tooley argues that since infants don't have the requisite cognitive capacities to have any interest in their continued life, they have no right to life, properly understood. Benjamin relies on similar premises to support the view that it is a "sentimental fiction" to suppose that saving an infant's life is something done on behalf of its own interests, and so the use of a best interest standard in life-and-death decisions about newborns is conceptually bankrupt.

Despite these arguments, many people believe deeply that infants do have a right to life (their killing is a crime against them, not only against their parents or the social order) and believe that we invest our energies and money in keeping them alive for their sakes, and not only ours. Given the tension between the principles and these moral convictions, what are our choices within a coherentist methodology? First, we can jettison these convictions, and by so doing achieve a greater coherence among our moral beliefs. Second, we can take the conflict with these beliefs to constitute a *reductio ad absurdum* of the principles, and be left with our moral views in their previous state of untidy disarray. Or, third, we may be content to let our convictions about infanticide simply remain as they are, a break in the web that may remain a trouble spot for the indefinite future, thus ensuring work, if not employment, for coming generations of moral philosophers.

The choice among these alternatives requires some evaluation of the elements to be traded off. How important and deeply held are our traditional convictions about infanticide? Are the other considered judgments that the principles systematize equally important to us, or should we be reconsidering our commitments to *them*? And given the stakes involved, how willing should we be to live with a little incoherence? So long as the norm of coherence is just one norm among others, we will, in other words, have to make a balancing judgment.

If, on the other hand, the norm of coherence is absolute or overriding, then the only option is to reject the stubborn convictions that are in the way. This is an unattractive alternative because it abandons the desirability of testing and justifying principles by appeal to actual moral convictions rather than appeal to abstract theory, one of the chief attractions of coherence views. It would also imply that a coherence theory of justification and a pluralist normative theory are incompatible, since by definition a pluralist system is composed of discrete and sometimes conflicting norms. The absolute demand for coherence would reveal an impulse to monism.

This defense of coherence models is defective for another reason. It will virtually never be the case that an offending considered judgment stands alone. It will connect in a host of ways to various moral principles and background theories, most likely different from those used to justify its rejection.

Concerning the wrongfulness of withholding treatment from the otherwise healthy elderly, for example, one might invoke a principle of equal respect for all persons, insisting that the lives of all persons are of equal value, and that scarce life-saving resources should be distributed by lot among them. This might be supplemented by a background theory that holds that the value of personal life consists in being able to appreciate one's life as a journey, in which goals are pursued and values sustained. The first would explain why it is *prima facie* wrong to withhold even scarce treatment purely on the basis of age. The second would explain, and perhaps more plausibly than Daniels is able to, why it would nevertheless be permissible to withhold treatment from his dying and demented aunt.

Of course, this is not an entirely unproblematic alternative. As should be apparent from the preceding example, it implies that there is no wrong done to them if life-saving treatment is withheld from infants, contrary to the convictions of common morality. In its favor, however, it accounts for our conviction that there is a greater imperative to provide an adult with a life-saving heart transplant than to perform life-saving fetal surgery—a conviction that Daniels' principle of equal opportunity does not recognize.[18]

The choice between these alternative sets of principles and judgments cannot be made solely on the basis of their degrees of coherence. Not only because there is no metric for "coherence." More importantly, the choice requires some judgment about the *moral significance* of the various elements that each set brings into coherence—how compelling are the principles and theories brought into play? how dear are the considered judgments that may have to be foregone? how much incoherence should we be willing to tolerate? These are judgments of moral weight, and the choice between the alternatives is, once more, a matter of balancing.

Can these unavoidable balancing judgments themselves be evaluated within a coherence model of justification? There are two reasons to think that this is not possible. First, these are not judgments *within* a system of principles, rules, and particular judgments. They are judgments *about* competing systems of principles, rules, and particular judgments. So their coherence would have to be judged relative to some meta-system of balancing judgments, about which the need for further balancing judgments would arise, and so on, leading to an infinite regress of spheres of justification. Second, such balancing judgments seem to be specific to the circumstances of the situation in which they are made, and can neither be stated as a rule or principle, nor derived from a rule or principle. If this is so, then no balancing judgment has implications for any other balancing judgment.

They don't exist as elements within a system of beliefs. In that case, they lie outside the possibility of coherence.

This means that Brink is wrong when he claims that in a coherence model of justification, justification is always inferential (Brink, 1989, p. 103) This is a critical difference he identifies between coherence models and intuitionism, since the latter holds that at least some justification is not inferential: some moral claims are self-evident or otherwise not subject to justification by appeal to further reasons. We've just seen, however, how arguments that appeal to coherence require balancing judgments whose warrant is not provided by coherence. Unless we can identify some other form of justification for these judgments, they mark the place where coherence models become intuitionistic.

The critical role played by balancing judgments also raises significant questions about the nature of the inference taken to be characteristic of a coherence model. Of course, many of the links that tie up the elements into a system are inferences of an ordinary kind: deductive inferences from theories to principles to considered judgments, or inductive inferences of various sorts that support factual generalizations or predictions. But what is the nature of the inference from *a set of claims about connectedness* among some parts of a system of beliefs to a claim about the truth of a particular assertion? This inference is neither deductive nor inductive; so what sort of inference is it? What positive description can we give of its features? Perhaps more importantly, by what standards can we judge the adequacy of such inferences?

These are questions seldom asked, let alone answered, in the literature advocating coherence models like wide reflective equilibrium.

For this reason, the ideal of wide reflective equilibrium does not provide any distinctive set of *standards* by which particular instances of moral reasoning are judged. It is instead a heuristic *model* for the construction of moral arguments, which drives reasoning toward consideration of the widest range of relevant considerations. The reasoning that is constructed in this process cannot be evaluated as a whole, but only piece by piece, using the critical tools already familiar to deductive and inductive logic, scientific hypothesis testing, and any other forms of inference that are relevant to claims about particular connections between parts of the belief system.

Thus, wide reflective equilibrium is not usefully thought of as an *alternative to* principle-based reasoning, case-based reasoning, or any of the other forms of reasoning that have been advocated within medical ethics and moral philosophy, and that will be discussed in chapters to follow. By definition, reasons always make connections between one belief and another, and so all forms of reasons have a place within a coherence model. But coherence could never substitute for these various ways of making connections, for without them there would be no glue binding the elements together into a system.

Summary

The discussion of the roles and limits of principles over the past two chapters points toward several tentative conclusions, which will need to be further elaborated and defended in what follows.

First, on a positive note, principles remain vitally important to reasoning in ethics, for all the reasons discussed in the previous chapter. They are a natural response to the demand for reasons so pertinent in ethics. They are useful in this role insofar as they help surface implicit assumptions as "hidden premises," or help to place a particular ethical question within a larger network of considerations, as in their use in wide reflective equilibrium. It seems implausible at this point that there could be any credible form of ethical reflection that did without principles altogether. We will, however, be considering some such usurpers later.

But it is also clear that appeals to principles cannot be the only form of justification needed for ethical deliberation, for this would make the problems of interpretation and conflicting principles unsolvable. The combination of Richardson's model of specification with the ideal of wide reflective equilibrium offers some partial solution to these problems, by suggesting that judgments about particular cases can help to justify an interpretation of a general principle. But although we have a good idea how to make inferences from general principles to particular cases, we don't have yet much idea how to make warranted inferences in this other direction. The ideal of wide reflective equilibrium suggests the possibility and the relevance of a wide variety of moral reasons that provide connections for our ethical thinking, but that work differently than the deductive inference upon which principled reasoning rests. What are these other types of reasons? What are their uses and limits? How are their uses connected with principle-based reasoning? Are each of these various sorts of reasons better suited for one kind of ethical question rather than another? These are all questions to be explored soon.

Another important conclusion of our discussion is that balancing judgments are unavoidable in any ethical argument that employs principles, whether they are used within a foundationalist or a coherence model of justification, with or without specification. What's more, these judgments are ones that seem to lie outside the mode of inference in which they are employed. They cannot be a matter of deduction from a set of higher-level principles, and neither are they judgments easily assimilated within a system of wide reflective equilibrium.

Does this mean such judgments must remain a matter of unprincipled moral intuition, as Richardson fears? If so, do they mark the boundary where reasoned ethical reflection stops? Or are there still ways in which such judgments might be critically evaluated, even if not inferentially justified? The ubiquity and necessity of judgment will only become more apparent in what follows.

Notes

1. See B. Andrew Lustig's 1992 article for more on this point.

2. Beauchamp and Childress do not explain just how this is accomplished in the face of the patient's direct question. For instance, does the physician say something like, "I can't really say for sure what the problem is until we repeat the test. Let's wait til then, when we can go over the results in detail." If the patient acquiesces in this plan, the case presents no ethical conflict with respect to autonomy. Alternatively, does the physician respond with a lie, like "I don't really see anything to worry about, but let's repeat the test just to make sure." Presumably, the balance of obligations could shift significantly if we add the obligation not to lie to the scales. A similar vagueness about practical details infects a number of their other illustrative cases, including the one that follows this case on the same page.

3. This reminds me of a joke told by Martin Benjamin: Tom Beauchamp is a utilitarian; Jim Childress is a Kantian. Beauchamp and Childress is an intuitionist.

4. Subsequent to the events Beauchamp and Childress describe, McAfee reversed his demands to discontinue his ventilator support after United Cerebral Palsy of Greater Birmingham and other disability advocacy groups offered him genuine alternatives to the hospitals and institutions in which he had resided or been treated (Herr, Bostrum and Barton, 1991, pp. 34–35).

5. See also Clouser and Gert (1990, p. 234).

6. See Lustig (1992, pp. 504–505) for a criticism similar to what follows (though he doesn't recognize that Beauchamp and Childress' account suffers from the same failing).

7. See Katz' 1984 discussion of the history and practice of disclosure in medicine.

8. For example, there is no reason to think that physicians, individually or as a group, could not meet the tests of universalizability and reversibility that Gert discusses (see esp. Gert, 1988, pp. 77–78).

9. This reasoning presumes that such blissful ignorance can be ensured by what the physician does or doesn't say. This presumption is surely false. But this is a very different criticism than the one Gert takes himself to be making.

10. Richardson's proposal was picked up by David DeGrazia (1992), who suggested that specification could help solve the problems plaguing Beauchamp and Childress' principlism. Beauchamp and Childress subsequently adopted DeGrazia's friendly amendment to their theory in the fourth edition of their book.

11. See, for example, Leon Kass' argument that because death annihilates the person to be benefitted, physician-aided dying cannot logically be thought to be beneficial to the patient (Kass, 1991, p. 474). Ironically, this form of argument was used first by the Stoics, but to reach the opposite conclusion: death cannot be a harm to the one who dies.

12. See Kuhn's discussion of the crisis faced by the phlogiston theory, one of the examples he uses to illustrate paradigm shifts in scientific theory (Kuhn, 1970, pp. 69–72).

13. See his various discussions of "reflective equilibrium" in *A Theory of Justice*: "justification is a matter of the mutual support of many considerations, of everything fitting together into one coherent view" (Rawls, 1971, p. 579).

14. The outline that follows is my own reconstruction of the argument that Daniels makes in this article, which on my reading can be easily recast into a model of wide reflective equilibrium. Daniels himself, however, never refers to his method in these terms.

15. Or the debate about the execution of Karla Fay Tucker, a woman convicted of viciously murdering two people, who on Texas' death row became a born-again Christian. See Verhovek (1998).

16. See Jecker (1991) for arguments against age-based allocation, which she thinks is especially problematic for women; and Cassel (1990), who objects to the generalizations regarding elderly patients that such policies rely upon.

17. See David DeGrazia's discussion (1991, p. 529).

18. See Kuhse and Singer (1988) for their argument against principles that seek to maximize life span.

Bibliography

Beauchamp, Tom L. and James F. Childress. 1994. *Principles of Biomedical Ethics*, 4th ed. New York: Oxford University Press.

Beauchamp, Tom L. and James F. Childress. 2001. *Principles of Biomedical Ethics*, 5th ed. New York: Oxford University Press.

Beauchamp, Tom L. and James F. Childress. 2009. *Principles of Biomedical Ethics*, 6th ed. New York: Oxford University Press.

Benjamin, Martin. 1983. "The Newborn's Interest in Continued Life: a Sentimental Fiction." *Bioethics Reporter: Ethical and Legal Issues in Health Care Administration and Human Experimentation*. Ed. James Childress et al. Frederick, MD: University Publications of America, Commentary 5.

Brink, David O. 1989. *Moral Realism and the Foundations of Ethics*. New York: Cambridge University Press.

Cassel, Christine K. 1990. "The Limits of Setting Limits." In *A Good Old Age: the Paradox of Setting Limits*, ed. Paul Homer and Martha Holstein. New York: Touchstone Books.

Clouser, K. Danner and Bernard Gert. 1990. "A Critique of Principlism." *Journal of Medicine and Philosophy* 15: 219–236.

Daniels, Norman. 1979. "Wide Reflective Equilibrium and Theory Acceptance in Ethics." *Journal of Philosophy* 76:256–282.

Daniels, Norman. 1987. "Equal Opportunity, Justice, and Health Care for the Elderly: A Prudential Account." In *Ethical Dimensions of Geriatric Care*, ed. Stuart F. Spicker, Stanley R. Ingman and Ian R. Lawson. Dordrecht: D. Reidel Publishing.

DeGrazia, David. 1992. "Moving Forward in Ethical Theory: Theories, Cases, and Specified Principlism." *Journal of Medicine and Philosophy* 17: 511–539.

Feinberg, Joel. 1974. "The Rights of Animals and Unborn Generations." In *Philosophy and Environmental Crisis*. Ed. William T. Blackstone. Athens: University of Georgia Press.

Gert, Bernard. 1988. *Morality: A New Justification of the Moral Rules*. New York: Oxford University Press.

Herr, Stanley S., Barry A. Bostrum and Rebecca S. Barton. 1992. "No Place to Go: Refusal of Life-Sustaining Treatment by Competent Persons with Disabilities." *Issues in Law and Medicine* 8: 3–36.

Jecker, Nancy S. 1991. "Age-Based Rationing and Women." *JAMA* 266:3012–3015.

Kass, Leon R. 1991. "Why Doctors Must Not Kill." *Commonweal* 118: 472–480.

Katz, Jay. 1984. *The Silent World of Doctor and Patient.* New York: The Free Press.

Kuhn, Thomas S. 1970. *The Structure of Scientific Revolutions,* 2nd ed. Chicago: University of Chicago Press.

Kuhse, Helga and Peter Singer. 1988. "Age and the Allocation of Medical Resources." *Journal of Medicine and Philosophy* 13: 101–116.

Lustig, B. Andrew. 1992. "The Method of 'Principlism': A Critique of the Critique." *Journal of Medicine and Philosophy* 17: 487–510.

Rawls, John. 1971. *A Theory of Justice.* Cambridge: Harvard University Press.

Richardson, Henry S. 1990. "Specifying Norms as a Way to Resolve Concrete Ethical Problems." *Philosophy and Public Affairs* 19 (Fall): 279–310.

Richardson, Henry S. 2000. "Specifying, Balancing, and Interpreting Bioethical Principles." *Journal of Medicine and Philosophy* 25: 285–307.

Tooley, Michael. 1985. *Abortion and Infanticide.* New York: Oxford University Press.

Verhovek, Sam Howe. 1998. "Karla Tucker is now gone, but several debates linger." *New York Times,* Feb. 5: A12.

Chapter 4

Casuistry: Ruled by Cases

Especially since the publication of *The Abuse of Casuistry*, by Albert R. Jonsen and Stephen Toulmin, many persons working in medical ethics have advocated the revival of the medieval art of casuistry as a method of moral thinking especially suited to addressing ethical problems in medicine. Given the frequency with which writers in medical ethics declare themselves casuists, there are still surprisingly few published attempts at any sustained, in-depth defense of the application of casuistical methods to specific problems in medical ethics.

In this chapter, I will argue that the appeal of casuistry is in many respects a superficial one that promises much more than it delivers. Despite the limitations I will identify, casuistry will still have some important roles to play in moral reflection.

The Appeal of Casuistry

Before beginning my critical assessment, it will be useful to get some understanding of why casuistry attracts such eager adherents from medical ethics. Understood vaguely as a method of moral reasoning rooted in judgments about cases rather than in commitments to abstract principles, casuistry's appeal has two sources—reactions against principle-based approaches to ethical problems, and the practical and pedagogical centrality of the "case" in medical ethics.

First, of course, many are attracted to casuistry because it seems to be a plausible alternative to principle-based approaches, which are suspect for all the sorts of reasons discussed in earlier chapters. There are two of these difficulties with principle-based approaches that casuistry aims particularly to avoid. One is the lack of consensus on any overarching ethical theory or principle. By relying instead on what seem to be firmer and more common agreements about particular paradigm cases of right and wrong, casuistry hopes to sidestep this difficulty with foundational approaches.

The other is the problem of interpretation of general principles that plagues their application to particular cases. As we've seen, one can't defend a specification of a general principle in its application to particular circumstances without relying on some intuitive balancing judgments. Since the casuist argues primarily from other *cases* rather than primarily from principles, the problem of interpretation would seem not to arise.

Casuistry is also attractive because in medical ethics the case is the central focus of professional attention. Cases are at the heart of teaching in medical ethics. Aside from a few anthologies, there's scarcely a textbook around that doesn't include a good supply of cases for students to gnaw on. The problems that are brought to the ethicist to solve are predominantly individual cases. And controversies and resolutions of controversy often turn around cases. A long line of cases served as successive focal points for arguments about the permissibility of withdrawing artificial food and fluids, which culminated in the Supreme Court opinion in the case of Nancy Cruzan (Annas, 1990).

Thus, a case-based method of reasoning seems just what the doctor ordered for medical ethics.

Casuistry to the Rescue?

At least for its modern exponents, casuistry fills that prescription. Although it makes use of moral rules, or maxims, these are more devices for organizing paradigmatic cases rather than independent and higher grounds of moral justification. Those grounds lie first and last in the paradigmatic cases that the maxims distill, and that embody our core moral beliefs.

When setting out to evaluate "casuistry," it is important to be precise about what we mean, since the term is used very loosely at times by those in medical ethics. "Casuistry" cannot usefully refer merely to the give-and-take of reasoned moral argument, and the resulting evolutionary improvement in moral understanding. Nor can it be a term applied whenever the circumstances of particular cases are thought to be ethically important.[1] Put so vaguely, there would be few moral philosophers, from utilitarians to deontologists, who wouldn't agree. If "casuistry" denotes anything distinctive here, it must be something in the special manner in which circumstances are employed or evaluated, not in the mere fact of their importance.

Neither can "casuistry" refer to the use of paradigm cases as a testing ground for the refinement of moral principles or theories. The use of paradigm cases may indeed be a feature of casuistry, but this alone does not distinguish it from other approaches to ethical reasoning.

For example, wide reflective equilibrium, discussed in the previous chapter, seeks to make use of moral consensus about paradigm cases ("considered judgments") in helping provide justification for ethical opinions. But there, the considered judgments are taken to play only an indirect role. Although they may motivate the refinement of general moral principles, they provide only some of the warrant for them. The principles within a wide reflective equilibrium are not taken merely to summarize a set of considered judgments.[2] General moral principles must also conform to the demands of various background theories, both moral and non-moral. Despite its use of paradigm cases or considered judgments, in wide reflective equilibrium it is principles that stand at the nexus of moral justification, with considered judgments playing a secondary, largely constraining role.

Jonsen and Toulmin provide a more precise definition of casuistry that helps to highlight its distinguishing characteristic. Casuistry is "the interpretation of moral issues, using procedures of reasoning based on paradigms and analogies, leading to the formulation of expert opinion about the existence and stringency of particular moral obligations, framed in terms of rules or maxims that are general but not universal or invariable, since they hold good with certainty only in the typical conditions of the agent and the circumstances of action" (Jonsen and Toulmin, 1988, p. 297).

In their book (Jonsen and Toulmin, 1988, Ch. 16), and in a later article by Jonsen alone (Jonsen, 1992), Jonsen and Toulmin further describe the characteristic steps in a casuistical analysis. The first task is to describe the problematic case in full detail, together with the moral reasons, or "maxims," that people would apply to the situation. This Jonsen calls the *Morphology* (Jonsen, 1992, pp. 298 ff.).

An adequate description of the case, and most especially the relevant maxims that would be applied to it, will make it possible for us next to place it into a *Taxonomy* identifying the "type" or types of case to which the problematic case belongs, and the paradigmatic examples of right and wrong conduct within the type (Jonsen, 1992, pp. 301 ff.).

One is now in the position to make the critical analogical judgment (rather than a deductive inference from a principle or rule) that assesses which of the paradigmatic cases most closely resembles the case under debate. This holistic judgment requires an appreciation of *Kinetics*: the "way in which one case imparts a kind of moral movement to other cases" (Jonsen, 1992, p. 303). One knows what that "movement" is by virtue of "practical wisdom." "Prudent judgment must discern the relevance of a maxim in the light of the matter under consideration" (Jonsen, 1992, p. 304).

The feature of casuistry that stands out as distinctive in Jonsen and Toulmin's characterization is its reliance on argument by analogy with paradigm cases. It is this feature that draws the important contrast with principle-based approaches, whose idealized mode of reasoning is a deductive inference from a well-specified principle to the case at hand.[3]

It is important to keep this contrast in mind, since it is easy to be misled by notions of "similarity" found in moral theory. Formal principles of justice and universality appeal to requirements to treat like cases alike, and one might infer from this that argument by casuistical analogy is inescapable in moral reasoning. James Childress, for example, points out that "one common statement of the formal principle of justice is 'treat similar cases in a similar way,'" and then infers that "this interpretation of justice requires. . . analogical reasoning" (Childress, 1990, p. S443). It may well permit analogical reasoning, but it doesn't require it. If one satisfies the requirement of the formal principle by appealing to a substantive principle of justice (e.g., Give first to the neediest), then two cases would be similar merely in the fact that they are both warranted by the principle. Analogical reasoning as Jonsen and Toulmin envision it is not a matter of deductive inference, but a matter of greater or lesser similarity, where even inconsistency can come in degrees.

Casuistry at Work: An Example

Carson Strong provides a more concrete picture of what this kind of reasoning looks like using an example of a Jehovah's Witness refusing a life-saving blood transfusion (although he doesn't use the Jonsen/Toulmin vocabulary) (Strong, 1988).

The problematic case is a pregnant, near-term Jehovah's Witness woman who developed abruptio placentae (premature separation of the placenta from the uterus), requiring a cesarean section to protect both mother and infant. She agreed to the cesarean section, but with no blood transfusion. Following surgery, which delivered a healthy child, she developed further complications, requiring blood transfusion to save her life. She continued to refuse blood, with the support of her husband, who said that if his wife died, he and other family could care for their seven children, despite their financial insecurity.

According to Strong, the maxims involved in this case are the principle of autonomy, which respects refusals of treatment by competent adults, in potential conflict with a principle of beneficence, which imposes a duty to protect the interests of the children in having their mother survive. Together with the description of the case, we would now have the Jonsen/Toulmin "morphology."

Corresponding to the alternative courses of action available (which in this case would be either to respect the woman's refusal, or not) we can identify paradigm cases that exemplify the circumstances in which the patient's right to autonomy is overcome by the obligation to protect her or her children's welfare, and the reverse. As one of his paradigmatic cases, Strong describes a Jehovah's Witness father refusing blood, who will leave no means of support, either financial or emotional, for his children after his death. In this case, Strong contends, the principle of beneficence rules, and a court order forcing treatment would be justified. The contrasting paradigmatic case would be one in which the Jehovah's Witness father is financially secure, with family members nearby. His surviving children will be easily and well supported if he should die. In this case, autonomy outweighs beneficence, and a court order would be unjustified.

We now have the problematic case placed within the Jonsen/Toulmin "taxonomy" and are ready to compare the actual case with the paradigmatic ones. The question will be which of the paradigm cases most closely matches the circumstances of the case being decided. This assessment of the "kinetics" of the cases is the judgment of "practical wisdom" that Jonsen refers to.

Strong's own judgment is that even though there are differences in "mitigating" factors, there is a "serious question" whether the family in the actual case could provide economic and emotional support for the deceased parent's children, just as there was in the first paradigmatic case. Therefore, Strong concludes, that paradigm case argues (by analogy) for the decision to seek a court order in the case at issue.

The Argument for Casuistry

What can be said on behalf of this approach to moral reasoning? Part of Jonsen and Toulmin's case is just to argue against the alternative, principle-based view, and so they echo many of the complaints against principle-driven ethics discussed earlier.

But they also have a positive argument that relies on a contrast they make (borrowed from Aristotle) between "theoretical" and "practical" knowledge. In reasoning theoretically, we are more certain of the truth of our axioms than of the conclusions reached by use of them (Jonsen and Toulmin, 1988, p. 25). In practical reasoning, it is the reverse. We are more certain that "Chicken is good to eat" than we are of any theoretical explanation or principle offered to support it.[4]

Their argument, then, is that ethical reasoning must also be practical rather than theoretical, since in ethics too we are much more certain about our judgments of particular cases than we are about any theoretical or general principle. If so, ethical thinking must be like other paradigmatic instances of "practical judgment." This conclusion is supported by features common to ethical thinking and other forms of practical reasoning: the arguments are concrete (about a specific case), temporal (in a specific historical context), and presumptive (their conclusions aren't necessarily or timelessly valid).

But merely to claim that ethical thinking is "practical" in these broad respects is not yet an argument on behalf of casuistry as the specific form that ethical thinking should take. (Note, for example, that utilitarian approaches can have all of the listed features of practical reasoning.) To make this additional argument, Jonsen and Toulmin place a lot of weight on the analogy between one form of practical judgment—medical diagnosis—and casuistry. Both rely on a holistic "pattern recognition" and arguments by analogy between "classical" or "paradigmatic" cases and a specific troubling case. If medical diagnosis exemplifies practical reasoning, and if ethical thinking is a kind of practical reasoning, then ethical thinking must look like medical diagnosis.

Presumably, Jonsen and Toulmin did not intend to make the argument quite this explicit, since the inference is logically fallacious.[5] Even in the form of an analogy, however, it still has significant problems as a positive argument on behalf of casuistry. Let's suppose that clinical diagnosis is a kind of pattern recognition, where one reasons by analogy from previous cases to make a diagnosis in the present one.[6] To begin, one important difference between ethical and diagnostic thinking is that the diagnostic judgment, unlike the ethical judgment, is not primarily a judgment about what to do. It's one thing to make the diagnostic judgment that your patient has benign prostatic hypertrophy, based on a holistic impression of the reported symptoms, the family history, the feel of the surface of the prostate on rectal exam, PSA levels, and so on. But it's a separate decision what to do about it: leave things alone, take a biopsy, perform surgery (but what sort?), treat symptomatically with drugs? This decision about action is not so easily thought to be a kind of pattern recognition where the decision is made by analogy with known cases. The decision about treatment (especially if one follows the decision analysts) is more a matter of toting up advantages and disadvantages of the alternatives, based on generalizations and probabilities, and basing one's final judgment on the weight of that evidence. Thus, if Jonsen and Toulmin had only taken the therapeutic judgment as their paradigm of practical reasoning, rather than the diagnostic one, the analogous model of ethical reasoning that would have emerged would look more like Beauchamp and Childress' balancing of competing ethical considerations than it would argument by analogy from paradigmatic cases.

Another significant problem arises from the claim that what diagnostic thinking and ethical thinking have in common is "pattern recognition." "Pattern recognition" is itself ambiguous as a description of a kind of judgment.

In one sense, pattern recognition is a holistic act of perception, where one either gets it, or doesn't. An experienced painter might hold up a chip of paint, compare it with a standardized color chart, and say, "Look, this is violet, not purple." But in another sense, pattern recognition is more like the recognition of consistency in reasoning. "Artificial insemination by donor is like adultery" is at its core more like an analytic judgment than a holistic perception, because it follows, and is sensitive to, an enumeration of the reasons that are thought to support the condemnation of adultery together with the evidence that many of these apply to the case of AID. Thus, to say that ethical thinking must be like diagnostic thinking because each of them involves "pattern recognition" begs the crucial question of which sort of pattern recognition is (or should be) used in ethics.

An important aspect of this distinction is that it is only the first sense of "pattern recognition" that supports thinking of ethical judgment as ultimately a matter of "discernment" by the expert, which Jonsen and Toulmin take to be an essential element of casuistry. If distinguishing right from wrong is like distinguishing violet from purple, there is no more gainsaying the judgment of the ethical expert than there is the judgment of the color expert. Indeed, since these judgments are acts of holistic and unanalyzable perception, we have to cede epistemic authority to someone in order to bring closure to disagreements, since by definition there would be no ways by which disagreements could be further understood and negotiated.[7] As others have noted (Juengst, 1989), there is a corresponding strain of moral authoritarianism in Jonsen and Toulmin's revival of casuistry, which is wholly consistent with casuistry's tradition.[8]

Problems and Limits of Casuistry

Even if the philosophical arguments on behalf of casuistry are not convincing, it might still be the case that in practice the casuistical model works as a satisfying, alternative framework for organizing our approaches to moral problems. But in fact there are serious limitations and objections even to its application. Indeed, what we find is that casuistry suffers from many of the same problems as principle-based approaches. This evaluation leaves open the possibility that casuistry may also offer some advantages, which can be employed without embracing casuistry as a wholesale alternative mode of justification. Before investigating this possibility, however, it is important to gain a fuller understanding of casuistry's limits.

Selecting the Paradigm Cases

First, note that any appeal to *a* set of "paradigm cases" assumes that the proper ones have been selected for comparison. In any contentious ethical question, however, where there are competing ethical considerations or "maxims," there will also be alternative sets of paradigm cases to which analogies can be drawn. Return, for example, to the case of the Jehovah's Witness woman discussed by Strong. Confronted with Strong's set of paradigmatic cases, she might well have asked in response whether he would have been prepared to remove a kidney from her without her consent, had one of her children needed a kidney transplant in order to get off dialysis. If the answer is "no" (which is the answer the courts have given), or even if it's "unsure," then isn't forced organ donation a paradigm case of a competing type that supports a decision *not* to transfuse her against her will, even for the sake of her children's health?

But now our casuistical reasoning is complicated by the need to decide from the very outset which of the two paradigmatic *types* is more compelling, and that judgment looks suspiciously just like a balancing between *prima facie* duties or principles. Which maxim takes priority: Parents have a duty not to harm their children? or Persons should not be forced to sacrifice themselves for others? Casuistry is not the superior alternative to a balancing approach. On the contrary, it too requires a balancing of moral weights between principles, or some alternative way of choosing between competing lines of paradigmatic cases before the analogical, casuistical part of the argument can even begin.

In a later article, Strong responded to this challenge by insisting that the case under contention is closer to his paradigm case than it is to a case of forced kidney donation. "In terms of casuistic factors, the case at hand is closer to my second case, for several reasons: having a kidney removed involves risks to health, whereas receiving a life-saving transfusion is medically beneficial; the potential harms to the pediatric renal patient can possibly be avoided by means other than forcibly removing a kidney from the mother, namely by receiving a kidney donated by someone else; and a transplant might not be successful, but the transfusion would be effective in saving the patient's life" (Strong, 1999, p. 410).

Note first that the paradigm case that I describe is a challenge to Strong's paradigm case itself, because my paradigm questions whether there can be *any* paradigm (i.e., incontestible) case of forced blood transfusion of parents for the sake of their surviving children.

Second, Strong's attempt to argue that the forced kidney donation case is too far removed from the circumstances of the Jehovah's Witness refusal does not succeed, because the cases are in fact closer than he claims. He suggests that the removal of a kidney imposes a harm on the patient, while transfusion provides a benefit. However, from the point of view of the Jehovah's Witness patient, the transfusion is at best a short-term benefit, exacted at the price of a long-term spiritual harm. Strong's attempt to distinguish the two cases implicitly relies upon one or another unargued assumption about how the benefit of the intervention is to be conceived: either that the patient's own values play no role in assessing that benefit, or that medical benefits are to be weighed more heavily than spiritual ones.

He also argues that there is an alternative available for the child needing a kidney transplant, namely finding another donor. But by analogy, there is an alternative available for the child facing the prospect of losing her mother, and in need of someone to serve as parent—namely, relying on the willingness of others in the community to serve as parent to the child.

Of course, in the last several paragraphs, I have been arguing casuistically, pointing out relevant analogies and disanalogies. But precisely because another line of cases has been brought into play, any ethical conclusion about the case in question has become more difficult, not less.

So, my criticism still stands. In any case where there is genuine moral conflict, there will be competing lines of paradigm cases, and casuistry as a method provides no warrant for a decision to turn to one set of paradigms rather than another.

Connecting Maxims and Paradigms to Cases

Second, it's not obvious how casuistry is any more articulate than a rule-based approach in explaining the connection between rules, principles, or maxims on the one hand, and specific moral judgments on the other, which in previous chapters is referred to as the problem of interpretation. Assume that the casuistical maxim is "Medical information should be kept confidential." According to the casuist, the meaning of that maxim is contained in a set of paradigmatic cases exemplifying when sharing information is a breach of confidentiality (e.g., when you tell the patient's husband that she has a lover), and when it's not (e.g., when you provide copies of records to the patient's insurance company with his written permission). So long as the case before us is exactly similar to one of the paradigmatic cases taken to exemplify the maxim, the application of the maxim to it is no problem. But what if the case before us is the decision by the patient's physician to ask a specialist to look over the patient's chart to provide help in diagnosing what may or may not be gall bladder trouble, but without getting the patient's explicit permission? Is that a breach of confidentiality or not? However one decides, there are no fully articulate grounds for the decision. On the one hand, the patient didn't give permission; on the other hand, it was done for the patient's benefit; on the one hand, for all we know the patient may have a deep distrust of strange consulting physicians; on the other hand, gall bladder disease is not a very stigmatizing ailment. This is precisely the spot where Jonsen and Toulmin resort to the mysteries of "discernment." Once outside the well-worn grounds of the paradigmatic cases, casuistry doesn't have the resources to explain why or to what extent the distinctive features of the non-paradigmatic case are determinative. As we have seen in earlier chapters, this is not a problem unique to casuistry; but casuistry doesn't seem to make any distinctive progress in solving it.

Carson Strong responds to this concern as well, arguing that "the claim that the case at hand is more like one paradigm than another can be articulated by pointing out the ways in which the casuistic factors in it are more similar to those of one paradigm than to the other" (Strong, 1999, p. 407).

Strong illustrates this with his casuistical analysis of the case of Pamela Hamilton, a 12-year-old who refused treatment for an osteosarcoma in her leg, based on religious beliefs shared with her parents. He bases his analysis on two putative paradigm cases of refusal of life-prolonging treatment for children. (In both of his cases, by the way, the patient has no significant degree of competency.) He then lists a variety of ways in which her case is like and unlike the two paradigm cases that he presents. He points out, for example, that "The probability that treatment would be effective in saving the patient's [Pamela's] life is slightly higher than the probability in case 3 [where it is assumed to be 15%], yet it is considerably lower than the probability in case 2 [assumed to be virtually 100%]" (Strong, 1999, p. 404).

At the end of his comparison, he concludes, "All things considered, the casuistic factors in case 1 are more similar to the factors in case 3 than they are to the factors in case 2, [hence] it is more reasonable to resolve case 1 in the manner that case 3 should be resolved than to resolve it in the manner that case 2 should be resolved" (Strong, 1999, p. 404).

The probability given for 5-year survival in case 3 is 15%; for Pamela Hamilton, Strong accepts that it might be as high as 50%. The question that is raised for Strong's comparison is why that isn't high enough to overcome parental objections. This is a critical question because surely there comes a point, as the chances for survival increase, where the moral judgment changes. Strong's method is based on the assumption of a kind of continuum, like the one that exists between black and white, and where I may be able to say that a particular shade of gray is closer to the black end than the white end of the continuum. But Strong's paradigm cases do not lie at opposite ends of a continuum like this. They are more comparable to the spectrum found between blue and green. We might be able to determine that a wavelength of radiation is closer in frequency to a green wavelength than a blue wavelength, but that won't tell us whether it is blue light or green light.

It is the same with Strong's method of argument. We may be able to judge that a given case lies closer to one paradigm than the other, but we don't know from that what side of the moral boundary it's on. Neither Strong's method, nor casuistry itself, can provide us a way of identifying where that point is that draws on reasons beyond the warrant of appeals to "discernment," "judgment," or "intuition." This is precisely the place where all casuists, including Strong, become intuitionists.

Ethical Blind Spots

A third difficulty for casuistry is its reliance on settled convictions about paradigm cases, where it runs the danger of uncritical conventionalism and conservatism. It seems to provide no way by which the settled paradigms themselves might be challenged. For this reason, even though casuists apply their art within a specific time and place, making no presumptions about "timeless" principles, casuistry is no more historically self-conscious than more "theoretical" approaches.

Finally, in its reliance on the paradigm case and argument by analogy, casuistry provides no avenue for other, indispensable types of moral argument, especially appeals to consequences. This is a liability that casuistry does not share with other approaches.

An Example: Jonsen's Casuistical Analysis of the "Case of Debbie"

All of these liabilities can be illustrated by Jonsen's application of the casuistical method to the well-known case of "Debbie."

"It's Over, Debbie" is a anonymously written short piece describing the actions of a gynecology resident called in the middle of the night to the room of a 20-year-old woman dying of ovarian cancer. She had not eaten or slept for days, was vomiting, and was suffering from pain and air hunger. Her only words to the resident were, "Let's get this over with." The resident asked the nurse to draw 20 mg of morphine, told the patient it would help her rest, and administered it, expecting that it would sufficiently depress her respiratory drive that she would quickly die. She did. (See Anonymous, 1988.)

The first step in the casuistical analysis of this case is to describe its "morphology": the circumstances of the case (the facts), and the maxims, or the pithy rules that seem to apply to the situation. In this case, the most obvious maxims that would be brought to bear are that (1) It is wrong to kill; (2) A physician should relieve pain and suffering; and (3) A physician should respect the patient's wishes regarding treatment, even when death may result.

The next step is to fit the case within a moral "taxonomy": identifying the "type" of case, and the paradigmatic examples of obviously right and wrong conduct within the type.

I argued earlier that this critical judgment is not itself amenable to casuistical reasoning. In his analysis, Jonsen stipulates that in Debbie's case, the type involved is cases of killing. In defending this judgment, he asserts that "the alternative proposal that the relevant taxonomy is care for the patient might be briefly entertained but would probably be dismissed by most commentators as question-begging" (Jonsen, 1992, p. 301).

Jonsen doesn't explain why placing the case in the taxonomy of care for the patient is any more question-begging than placing it in the taxonomy of killing, when the question seems precisely to be which of these competing moral imperatives should govern our moral judgment about this case. The lack of an explanation is not surprising, because the casuistical argument by analogy cannot adequately handle this sort of question.

Argument by analogy is directed to answering the question, "Is Debbie's case more like paradigmatic cases of killing, or paradigmatic cases of caring, or paradigmatic cases of respecting refusals of life-saving treatment?" When faced with a genuine moral problem, the answer to this question is going to be "A little bit of each." We can't categorically classify the case as only one or the other "type." So we are pushed onto a different kind of question, which is not a question of *classification*, but of moral weight: in the circumstances, which of these maxims is the more important to follow? The question, and its answer, are the staples of Rossian balancing of conflicting obligations. The answer, admittedly, is a judgment that may be relative to the circumstances of the case. It is not a judgment, however, that can be adequately based on analogies with paradigm cases, unless we already have at hand a paradigmatic case that is just like the present one, and that exemplifies an already well-accepted balancing of the competing considerations. But in that instance, we wouldn't be having a moral controversy about the case before us!

Another limitation of casuistry, which may be unique to it, is its inability to account for one of the major kinds of reasoning applied to the issue of voluntary active euthanasia: appeals to the consequences of any policy permitting active euthanasia.

In his discussion of the case, Jonsen asserts that an "approach that the casuist might take is to explore the implications of a physician accepting voluntary euthanasia requests even in appropriate circumstances. . . this approach is a form of the so-called 'slippery slope' response" ([9], Jonsen, 1992, p. 305).

The argument is a familiar one: if we permit physicians to provide active euthanasia to patients at their request, we will be launched on a slippery slope that leads to the horrors of the Nazi "euthanasia" program. This is not an analogical argument. Assessment of it turns on an evaluation of the strength of the factual evidence that this would indeed be the consequence of permitting active euthanasia. No doubt a casuist, like any other moral thinker, should take account of potential consequences of policies or patterns of choices, but this critical evaluation lies outside the bounds of case-focused casuistical thinking. And naturally, the Nazi program should be taken as a paradigmatic case of an evil euthanasia policy. But a slippery slope argument does not usually assert that voluntary euthanasia requests even in appropriate circumstances are morally just *like* a Nazi program, but rather that they may *lead to* an evil program. Such an argument would rely on the decidedly non-casuistical (and false) principle that whatever practices may lead to an evil are themselves evil.

Another characteristic problem surfaces even if we allow by stipulation that the case of Debbie is properly classified as a killing, rather than as some other type of act. According to the method of casuistry, our job would be to see how this case fits into the taxonomy of paradigmatic cases involving killing: unprovoked wanton killing, killing for personal gain, killing in a jealous rage, killing in self-defense, killing to protect others, etc., all of which offer elaborations of what we mean by the maxim "Thou shall not kill."

Jonsen's assessment is that "The fact that [paradigmatic] exceptions to the prohibition against killing remain very close to the protection of self and others suggests that killing to relieve pain [or with consent] might be an inadequate candidate" for being classified as a justifiable killing (Jonsen, 1992, p. 302).

Here we confront one of the other fundamental problems with casuistry—its uncritical conventionality. The method assumes that everything that might be relevant to justifying a killing has already been incorporated into the settled, conventional paradigms. The reliance on analogies with those conventional paradigms cannot answer what is perhaps the critical moral question raised by voluntary euthanasia: is consent a morally valid exception to the prohibition against killing? The standard paradigms beg this question, because they never have taken it up (or else they answer it dogmatically).

There is an historical reason for this. The idea that my life may be at my own disposal, rather than God's, is of only recent vintage. If the wrongness of killing is thought to consist in the usurpation of God's prerogative, then my consent to my own death is of course beside the point. If it hadn't been for the role of Middle Eastern theology in European moral development, the paradigms of justified killing might have been quite different.

As a method of moral analysis, casuistry can neither recognize this historical contingency, nor accept the moral relevance of any theological or other critique of it, which would be critiques of a non-casuistical sort. In this respect, the casuistical evaluation of voluntary euthanasia is no more historically aware than principle-based approaches would be.[9]

Finally, to complete our illustrations of casuistry's limitations, we should take a look at Jonsen's resolution of the case, which assesses its "kinetics":

> "In Debbie's case, the degree of her lucidity, the extent of her pain and its intractability, the scope of the resident's familiarity with her case, are all crucial features... susceptible of greater and less and the only way of judging 'how great and how less' comes from the wisdom of experience... Debbie's case is resolved casuistically with ease... the casuist can note that defects in the voluntary nature of the request... are sufficiently serious that no exception to the dominance of the maxim against killing is justified. The resident was wrong to administer the morphine in a lethal dose."
>
> (Jonsen, 1992, pp. 304–306)

There are two aspects of this reasoning that are significant for the evaluation of casuistry. First, the judgment that her request was not sufficiently voluntary is not based on any casuistical argument by analogy to any paradigm of justified killing, even though Jonsen has said that this is the pertinent classification. For by his admission, there are no accepted paradigm cases of ethically justifiable voluntary euthanasia.

At best, Jonsen is making his casuistical assessment relative to paradigms of acceptable refusals of life-prolonging treatment. But if these cases are the pertinent analogues, then Jonsen's conclusion about Debbie's case will not come as easily as he claims. When the question is whether to accept a patient's refusal of a life-prolonging treatment, the level of evidence for her competency that's demanded is usually taken to be relative to the price that will be paid if an incompetent refusal is in fact mistakenly

honored (see Buchanan and Brock, 1989, Ch. 1). If in the circumstances, the harm to the patient of withholding the treatment is
small, the standard of evidence will be low. Thus, in Debbie's case,
the question would be whether we should have honored her
demand not to be placed on a respirator, if she had made it under
the same problematic conditions as her apparent request for
active euthanasia. I am confident the answer is "Yes;" at the very
least, it is not an easy "No." But then, an argument by analogy
would appear to support a judgment about the case opposite to
the one favored by Jonsen.

We have here an illustration of yet another of the liabilities of
casuistry mentioned earlier. The moral judgment that we reach
by way of casuistical analogy will depend mightily on which type
of paradigm case we take to be the right analogue. That choice, in
turn, cannot itself be one that is based on analogies to paradigm
cases.

A final limitation revealed by Jonsen's conclusion is that in
making the judgment that Debbie's request was not sufficiently
voluntary, the casuist is really in no better shape than adherents
of a principle-based approach, who also must judge whether a
principle supporting voluntary euthanasia for the competent
informed adult applied in this case or not. The casuist, relying as
he does on the deliverance of "practical wisdom" rather than on
any further reasoning, analogical or otherwise, is no more articulate than anyone else in explaining the connection between the
maxim or principle and its application to any non-paradigmatic
case at hand.

What Can Be Salvaged?

Casuistry is promoted as an antidote to the serious inadequacies
that plague the dominant principle-based approach in medical

ethics. A principle-based approach seems unable to avoid the necessity of relying on intuitive judgments in balancing competing ethical principles; it cannot adequately support the interpretations and judgments that must be made in applying principles to cases; it may be naive about its own historical contingency; and it gives principles an epistemological pride of place over concrete judgments of cases that they don't deserve.

Except perhaps for the last of these, however, we've just seen how casuistry suffers from the very same, or closely related, difficulties. It has, in addition, its own special problems, most importantly an inherent moral conservatism that seems inadequate for handling the sorts of unprecedented ethical issues that are arising in health care.

Casuistry, therefore, is by no means an alternate model of moral reasoning preferable or superior to principle-based approaches in medical ethics. And yet casuistry's starting premise—that our understanding of our moral principles is rooted in paradigmatic cases—is nevertheless appealing. Casuistical analysis, in the most general sense of drawing comparisons with paradigmatic cases, may still be a useful element of moral problem-solving. What more modest purposes might it serve? I think there are several.

Paradigm Cases as Tools of Ethical Discovery

To begin with, determining whether the problem case fits closely with a paradigmatically right or wrong action is an essential first step in understanding the nature of the moral issue it presents. It may be that when fully and properly described, the case is not morally problematic at all, because the right action is patently clear, and no further analysis or argument is called for.

For example, it would make a difference to our ambivalence about the case of Debbie if it turned out that she and the resident were deep and bitter enemies, for then there would be reason to worry that the resident's motives were in part malevolent. This would be because the case would now much more closely resemble some paradigmatic cases of wrongful killing. These paradigm cases would at least alert us to the moral relevance of this new factor, even if by itself it was not a decisive one.

They would also provide alternative frameworks from which to explore reinterpretations of the events of the case, which would aim to determine whether this was itself a paradigm case of wrongful killing. We would, for example, now have reason to reinterpret what Debbie meant when she told the resident, "Let's get this over with."

One way to put this is to say that paradigm cases can point to some of the ways the story about the present case needs to be filled out before we can make an adequately informed judgment about the nature of the moral problem that faces us. Did the resident commit a plain, old-fashioned murder, or not? Casuistical appeal to paradigm cases can help us investigate and answer that question. If the conclusion is that the resident committed something very like a murder, that's ethically important. Then, for example, we would know that this is a matter for the prosecutor rather than the philosopher. If the conclusion is that the resident committed something significantly unlike a murder, then we know that we have a more difficult ethical judgment to make, and knowing that is also helpful. Casuistry, however, will not be of much further assistance in making that more uncertain judgment, for the reasons discussed in this chapter.

This suggests that analogies with paradigm cases are most useful as a tool of ethical investigation applied to enrich our moral understanding of particular cases. But couldn't such analogies be of similar help with more general ethical questions, such as those presented by policy disputes? I think the answer may be "No," for reasons that can be drawn from a couple of examples.

Analogies Not Useful for Assessing Social Consequences

Take first an analogy frequently used in the debate about the use of fetal tissue obtained from aborted fetuses. One of the questions posed in that debate is whether the use of such tissue by physicians and their patients makes them complicit in the abortions that produced it. An analogy is often used to argue that the use of fetal tissue implies no complicity in abortion: It is not uncommon, and it is clearly morally acceptable, to obtain organs from victims of murder who die while on life support in the hospital. No one thinks that the use of these organs implies any approval of murder, or mitigates the wrongfulness of murder, or encourages murderers. And so by analogy, even if we assume that abortion is the moral equivalent of murder, the use of organs or tissues from murdered fetuses carries no taint of complicity in the immoral act.

The use of organs from murder victims is a paradigm case of when one may benefit from an immoral action without being complicitous in it, and the casuistical question would be whether the use of tissue from aborted fetuses is sufficiently like the paradigm case. As Lynn Gillam (1997) points out, there are a number of significant disanalogies. Most importantly for my purposes, the disanalogies she identifies are rooted in the fact that we already have in place an entrenched set of intuitions and social practices about the wrongfulness of murder, which aren't present in the case of abortion—that is, we're all agreed that garden-variety murders are wrong; we have no such agreement about abortion.

This difference in social attitudes and practices opens up avenues of social causation that attach to the use of organs from aborted fetuses and not to the use of organs from murder victims. For example:

"it seems quite plausible that beliefs about the wrongness of abortion may be undermined by the use of fetal tissue... It may be thought, for example, that 'doctors would not use this tissue if they really thought that abortion was wrong,' or 'abortion can't be so bad if it can help people with terrible diseases like Parkinson's."

(Gillam, 1997, pp. 405–406)

The superficial retort is to ask why people might think such things about abortion when no such thoughts occur to them regarding the murders that lead to organ donation. The answer is that the condemnation of murder is so deeply embedded in our moral attitudes that the idea that its wrongfulness might be mitigated by the practice of organ donation is simply beyond the pale. Not so regarding abortion, where there is no well-settled moral view and where people's moral attitudes are more pliable. Thus the use of fetal tissue from abortions raises the possibility of social consequences that the use of organs from murder victims does not, precisely because only the latter rests within a settled paradigm around which social and attitudinal boundaries have formed. The original question about the moral taint of fetal tissue transplantation cannot be settled by an argument from analogy, but only by empirical study of the actual social consequences of the practice.

What this example suggests is that there may be a systematic, if not universal, difficulty in using arguments by analogy from paradigm cases to address ethical issues of policy. Issues of policy are sensitive to the possible consequences and social ramifications of instituting a new practice, which are always relevant even when not decisive. But paradigm cases, precisely because they are already embedded in a matrix of moral and social institutions different than those that might surround the policy or practice under dispute, may be either misleading or uninformative regarding the critical questions about consequences.

Analogies Must Be Tested by Principle

Another limitation of argument by analogy regarding questions of policy is that disputes about the analogies will need to be settled by some appeal to principle.

Take the sort of example mentioned earlier: the analogy drawn between forced organ donation, and forced blood transfusion or forced cesarean section. If the first is morally prohibited despite the good that might sometimes be done by it, so surely are the others.

Of course, if forced blood transfusions or cesarean sections are really morally contentious issues, the argument won't go so easily. Those who think they are sometimes justifiable will want to claim that there are significant disanalogies between some instances of these practices and forced organ donation. When they do so, how could these disanalogies be evaluated?

One answer is suggested by James Childress' discussion of the case of A.C., a dying and finally comatose woman whose premature child was delivered by cesarean section without explicit consideration of her wishes. The appellate court that eventually heard the case sided with the view that the lack of any attempt to get her consent or ascertain her wishes by substituted judgment made this intervention ethically and legally illegitimate. The majority opinion made explicit use of the analogy with forced organ donation.

Childress focuses his discussion on the minority opinion written by Judge Belson, who argues against the majority view by identifying a number of disanalogies between the situation of a pregnant woman like A.C. and the sorts of cases in which forced organ donation has been rejected. For example, Belson points to:

> "the singular nature of the dependency of the unborn child upon the mother. A woman carrying a viable unborn

child is not in the same category as a relative, friend, or
stranger called upon to donate bone marrow or an organ
for transplant."

(in Childress, 1990, S445)

Belson is responding in kind, using argument by disanalogy to
refute the analogical argument employed by the majority. The
critical question for his argument is whether this difference, as
well as the others he identifies, is an ethically significant one.
And the critical question for the use of casuistry as a method in
policy disputes is whether argument by analogy can address
these questions of significance.

The strategy employed by Childress in his analysis of Belson's
arguments suggests that the questions of significance raised
by argument by analogy are not answered by recourse to more
argument by analogy. Childress responds to Belson:

"it is unclear why a mother (or father) shouldn't be ordered
to provide bone marrow, or perhaps even a kidney, if a caesarian section is justified. After all, ... even though the
child now exists in physical independence, it may depend
on the mother for survival in the absence of any other
compatible donors for an organ (perhaps a portion of a
liver) just as much as the unborn child."

(Childress, 1990, pp. S445–446)

The strategy is to abstract out a principle from the claimed
significance of the analogical factor under question, and then
test the principle against paradigm cases or considered judgments. Belson's analogical argument is taken to rely on a principle to the effect that where there is a high degree of dependency,
there is a duty of those depended upon to provide needed
aid. Taking previous court decisions regarding forced organ

donations as paradigms, Childress shows that this principle is false, and concludes that Belson has not established (and maybe cannot establish) that the difference he relies on is morally significant.

This strategy is not analogical, and is in fact antithetical to argument by analogy. An argument by analogy places importance on matters of degree; reliance on principles necessarily obscures such differences. Belson's argument rests on a claim for the significance of the uniquely intimate degree of dependency of fetus on mother. Childress' response has to rely upon a principle regarding dependency under which other cases, involving some lesser degree or different type of dependency, can be subsumed.

There is a sense in which this sort of critical evaluation systematically begs the question against arguments by analogy, but it may be an unavoidable question-begging. Childress' argument must assume that the very particular degree or type of dependency that Belson thinks is significant is not so. But what other form of argument could there be that had any chance of getting beyond bare conflict between different intuitions or "discernments" about the significance of the analogical factors employed?

There are no obvious alternatives to the employment of principle in evaluating analogical arguments, at least when dispute remains regarding the significance of the analogies employed. For this reason, we should conclude that casuistry and argument by analogy offer limited help in evaluating conflicting positions on matters of policy in medical ethics.

Summary

Although much more problematic than often appreciated, casuistry may still be a useful tool for ethical investigation regarding specific cases in medical ethics, even if its worth as a method of justification or critical evaluation of contested choices remains under question. When it comes to policy questions, casuistry cannot make the assessment of consequences that is so essential to the evaluation of policy. Arguments by analogy are often employed in legal and policy debates, where they can usefully draw our attention to the most ethically salient factors needed attention. They cannot, however, assess whether any particular similarity or difference found with paradigm cases is ethically dispositive. For that, we seem driven back to the use of principles.

Notes

1. Jonsen, for example, points out that "when we ponder particularly difficult cases, circumstances loom large," and can make a significant difference in our moral evaluation. The "evaluation of circumstances," he suggests, is the particular province of casuistry (Jonsen, 1995, p. 243).

2. See Daniels (1979) for the distinction he makes between a "narrow" and a "wide" reflective equilibrium. He rejects the former as too susceptible to an uncritical relativism.

3. In another article, Jonsen makes this even plainer: "[Within casuistry] ethical reasoning is primarily reasoning by analogy, seeking to identify cases similar to the one under scrutiny and to discern whether the changed circumstances justify a different judgment in the new case than they did in the former" (Jonsen, 1995, p. 245).

4. Parenthetically, this is a badly ambiguous example for Jonsen and Toulmin to use, even if we should excuse the Greeks for it. Clearly, whether their claim is true or not depends on whether we understand the example to mean "Chicken tastes good when eaten" or "Chicken is a healthy food to eat." Only the first is more secure than any theoretical explanation or justification for it; but presumably Jonsen and Toulmin don't want to assimilate ethical judgments to matters of taste.

5. It would be like saying that since a sparrow is a bird and a penguin is a bird, sparrows must look like penguins, a conclusion whose small (generic) grain of truth is little compensation for its gross misrepresentation.

6. Although one should note that this model of diagnostic thinking is itself a matter of contention. Attempts to computer-model diagnosis, for example, assume that the process is implicitly Bayesian.

7. Of course, there is another reason we cede epistemic authority to experts: we haven't the time to become experts ourselves, and the experts' past performance has shown their judgments to be reliable ones. We trust the uncanny diagnostician because time and time again, he has turned out to be right. But this is not an explanation useful for Jonsen and Toulmin. Outside the mantle of religious authority, there is no comparable method of confirmation available for judging the trustworthiness of the ethical expert. (I'm grateful to Ed Erde for reminding me of this alternative.)

8. See my brief exploration of casuistry's history for elaboration of this point, in Tomlinson, 1994, pp. 12–13.

9. In a later article, Jonsen concedes that this may be a limitation of casuistry, the correction of which will require recourse to moral principle and theory. But then he tries to blunt the impact of this criticism by characterizing casuistry in a way that has it refer simply to the give-and-take of moral argument (see Jonsen, 1995, pp. 246 ff.).

Bibliography

Annas, George J. 1990. "Nancy Cruzan and the Right to Die." *New England Journal of Medicine* 323:670–674.

Anonymous. 1988. "It's Over, Debbie." *JAMA* 259:272.

Boyle, Joseph. 1991. "Who Is Entitled to Double Effect?" *Journal of Medicine and Philosophy* 16:475–494.

Buchanan, Allen E. and Dan W. Brock. 1989. *Deciding for Others: The Ethics of Surrogate Decision Making.* Cambridge: Cambridge University Press, Ch. 1.

Childress, James F. 1990. "Analogical Reasoning: Organ/Tissue Donation and Caesarian Sections." *Biolaw* 2:S443–447.

Daniels, Norman. 1979. "Wide Reflective Equilibrium and Theory Acceptance in Ethics." *Journal of Philosophy* 76:256–282.

Gillam, Lynn. 1997. "Arguing by Analogy in the Fetal Tissue Debate." *Bioethics* 11:397–412.

Jonsen, Albert R.1992. "Casuistry as Methodology in Clinical Ethics." *Theoretical Medicine* 12:295–308.

Jonsen, Albert R. 1995. "Casuistry: An Alternative or a Complement to Principles?" *Kennedy Institute of Ethics Journal* 5:237–251.

Jonsen, Albert R. and Stephen Toulmin. 1988. *The Abuse of Casuistry: A History of Moral Reasoning.* Berkeley: University of California Press.

Juengst, Eric T. 1989. "Casuistry and the Locus of Certainty in Ethics." *Medical Humanities Review* January:19–27.

Quill, Timothy E. 1991. "Death and Dignity: A Case of Individualized Decision Making." *New England Journal of Medicine* 324:691–694.

Sommerville, Johann Peter. 1988. "The "New Art of Lying": Equivocation, Mental Reservation, and Casuistry." In *Conscience and Casuistry in Early Modern Europe*, ed. Edmund Leites. Cambridge: Cambridge University Press: 159–184.

Strong, Carson. 1988. "Justification in Ethics." In: B. A. Brody, ed. *Moral Theory and Moral Judgments in Medical Ethics.* Dordrecht: Kluwer, 193–211.

Strong, Carson. 1999. "Critiques of Casuistry and Why They Are Mistaken." *Theoretical Medicine and Bioethics* 20:395–411.

Tomlinson, Tom. 1994. "Casuistry in Medical Ethics: Rehabilitated or Repeat Offender?" *Theoretical Medicine* 15:5–20.

Tomlinson, Tom. 1998. "Why the Critiques of Casuistry Still Stand." Unpublished manuscript.

Chapter 5

Narrative Ethics

The Uses of Stories[1]

Stories are everywhere in the practice of health care. They are often compelling stories, too, whether they are tragic or triumphant. We make hit TV shows out of them, from *Dr. Welby* to *House*.

What might stories provide for us besides the pleasure of reading and telling them? Could they deepen our understanding of ethical problems and choices? This is a live question in large part because, as we have seen, principle-based and analytical modes of ethical reflection have come under increasingly skeptical scrutiny. The problem of interpretation and the problem of balancing competing ethical considerations linger as obstacles to giving a solely principle-based account of ethical reflection. Perhaps stories offer the additional resources we need. The problem of interpretation, for example, is that in their abstractness, high- or even medium-level ethical principles are too removed from and insensitive to the specifics of the very particular living cases to which they are "applied." Analogously, the problem of balancing may be most difficult when it is posed as a conflict between abstract values (e.g., autonomy vs. benevolence), when it is hard for us to have a keenly felt understanding of what is at stake in the choice between them. By contrast with systems of moral principles, stories are all about particular people, places, and events. If abstractness is the problem, stories (or "narratives") would seem to be part of the solution. And so "narrative ethics" is born.

Sounds pretty reasonable . . . in the abstract. When we get down to specific claims and arguments concerning just how narrative might contribute to reasoned ethical reflection, however, the water becomes a good deal murkier.

Before descending for a closer look, it will be helpful to make some distinctions. First, let's distinguish two different roles commonly envisioned for narratives in health care ethics. The first sees stories playing a part in general moral or professional development. The reading and study of stories, it is said, has salutary effects on moral development through the enhancement of perceptiveness, sensitivity, sympathy, or other virtues. This claim will not be the focus of my attention here. Before setting it aside, I'll just note that my more literary acquaintances are nice to sit down with for a chaw and a chat, but I can't say that I've noticed any generally higher level of ethical acumen or comportment among them.[2]

It is the second role for narrative that interests me more, and is more germane to the themes of this book. This sees narrative serving a central epistemic function in the discovery, justification, or application of ethical knowledge—a role that fills the gaps inherent in any analytical, rule-based method. What is that epistemic role? How does it work? Why should we have confidence in it?

There are a variety of answers given to these questions, and they can be sorted on the basis of another set of distinctions: whether the stories are received (read, viewed, or heard) or created (written, told, or enacted).[3] In what follows, I will argue that stories we create are more fruitful for ethical knowledge than those we receive; but even so, those do little to replace reliance on principle or remedy the limits of principle-based reflection.

Literature and Moral Knowledge

One of the most common claims is that reading stories can enlarge our base of morally relevant knowledge. This idea is expressed in a variety of ways.

> "It is the precise role of narrative to offer us ways of experiencing [the] effects [of destructive alternatives] without experimenting with our own lives as well."
>
> (Burrell and Hauerwas, 1977, p. 138)

A novel like *David Copperfield* can "enlarge the moral imagination" in a way that "makes plain [the moral] cost" of a set of beliefs, attitudes, or policy. Dickens does this not so much by presenting facts hitherto unknown, but by doing so in a way that "engages" us so that we are brought to care about them (Diamond, 1982, p. 33).

The reading of literature provides "vicarious experience [which serves] as a means of sympathetically participating in the lives of others. . . By cultivating experience through imagination, through metaphor, through creative reading, a bridge can be established between the world of the patient (the other) and the world of the nurse or the physician or ethicist (the self)" (Radey, 1992, p. 40).

So long as we don't press any questions about how this role is to be played in the context of medical ethics, all of this seems innocuously and vaguely true. For the Victorian distant in space and class from the people of Dickens' world, a novel like *David Copperfield* or *Hard Times* may perhaps have been the best and certainly the most agreeable way to gain some sympathetic understanding of people who were otherwise alien to the reader.

But reading stories is not the only and may not be the best way to enlarge our understanding of people we don't know. Couldn't we do so by working with them, sharing experiences with them (real, not vicarious), talking with them? Isn't this in fact the way that we most commonly improve upon our understanding of others?

To put this question into the context of medical practice, isn't it by talking to the actual patient, seeing his real suffering, feeling sympathy for his genuine plight, that we cross Radey's bridge between the patient on the one side and the doctor, nurse, or ethicist on the other? A vicarious literary experience or secondhand story would be a poor substitute.

Of course I recognize that no one would advocate wholesale substitution of literary experiences for real ones. Rather, we should think of the stories we might read as useful *supplements* to our understandings of patients. Even this more modest suggestion raises an important difficulty. As all advocates of narrative ethics observe, a good story is about a very particular set of circumstances inhabited by characters with specific and unique histories, identities, and trajectories. But then how will even a very good story, even a very good story about a person in circumstances just like my patient's, provide me with useful and accurate insights about that real person's feelings, motives, or outlook? Well, perhaps the story will suggest to me some of the ways that a person in such circumstances may respond, and then I can explore those possibilities with my patient.

So the story can illustrate some general truths about human nature, which I may then tentatively apply to particular situations before me? This is no doubt true of many good stories, but this feature would not distinguish narrative ethics from other modes of moral knowledge. Remember that the special virtue of narrative, the mark that would distinguish it from the arid abstractions of ethics engineering, is that it remains in the world of the particular. Which kind of knowledge about patients *is* provided in stories—knowledge of the particular or knowledge of the general?

Neither choice is a comforting one for the claim that the read story provides a special source of morally relevant knowledge, useful for deliberating about real people's lives. For if the truth of the story is truth only for the characters portrayed in it, then it tells me nothing directly about those who don't live in that particular story. And if the truth of the story is alleged to be truth for all similarly situated, then the deliberately constructed particulars of the story provide scant evidence by themselves that the character is truly Everyman. Novels and stories become at best vivid illustrations of knowledge to be verified through other means.

None of this is to say that stories could not be a valuable source of moral sentiments. Diamond comes closest to the humble truth when she points out that what is notable about Dickens' art is not the presentation of facts, like a tract from some 19th-century Children's Defense Fund, but the creation of fellow-feeling in the reader. That feeling is morally animating, and the having of it may be indispensable to moral judgment. Reading, seeing, or hearing a story is one way to get that feeling. But the feeling can't be morally warranted merely by the fact that a story creates it. Readers of *Hard Times* may carry away one sort of moral attitude toward the poor and marginalized; readers of Ayn Rand's *Atlas Shrugged* another; and readers of William L. Pierce's notorious *The Turner Diaries* yet another. The fact is, unless we assume that the writers of stories have a special moral wisdom, we must make an independent judgment of the morality implicit in their work. Some works of fiction will be morally exemplary; some will be contemptible; most will be a mixed bag that will require us to bring skills and standards of ethical judgment to the work.

This does not mean that stories can't serve to challenge the moral assumptions we bring to them, and so initiate a rethinking of those assumptions. As Martha Nussbaum points out, Dickens' *Hard Times* is a sustained indictment of the view that the general welfare is all morality aims at, and that it is to be understood as nothing more than the aggregation of individual self-interest (Nussbaum, 1995, esp. the chapters on "The Literary Imagination" and "Fancy"). It is clear that novels can be written, and read, as critiques (or celebrations) of various moral points of view. But in no case are they likely to succeed in that purpose by themselves. In large part, this is because their success in eliciting the intended response on the part of the reader depends on the reader already having the moral dispositions the novel hopes to awaken or rely upon. Without them, she is not only unlikely to respond sympathetically to the novel's characters or to recognize its moral force; she's also unlikely to read it at all! Imagine a Mr. Gradgrind, the mercilessly utilitarian Member of Parliament in the novel, reading *Hard Times*; it's implausible to suppose he would appreciate its moral lessons in the same way Martha Nussbaum does. Perhaps the reading of a story could play some part in shifting moral opinion, but it could only be in conjunction with the use of other tools, like appeals to systematic moral analysis and theory.

Stories are often problematic teachers of moral lessons for another reason: they are written from a point of view, and for the purpose of vividly communicating that point of view. The result will be that certain aspects of the moral situation will be emphasized at the expense of others; a story that dutifully neglected nothing of possible moral relevance would have no point of view at all. This artistic selectivity can lead to a kind of ethical hyperbole that obscures or neglects complexities that would be inimical to the intended portrayal. Nussbaum's discussion of *Hard Times* provides an example of this.

Sissy Jupe is the warmly human heroine of the novel, and serves as the contrast against which its other coldly utilitarian characters are judged. Nussbaum notes the way Sissy's naive compassion rebukes complacent utilitarian calculation:

> "Sissy is told by her utilitarian teacher that in 'an immense town' of a million inhabitants only twenty-five are starved to death in the streets. The teacher, M'Choakumchild, asks her what she thinks about this—plainly expecting an answer expressing satisfaction that the numbers are so low. Sissy's response, however, is that 'it must be just as hard upon those who were starved, whether the others were a million, or a million million.' Again, told that in a given period of time a hundred thousand people took sea voyages and only five hundred drowned, Sissy remarks that this low percentage is 'nothing to the relations and friends of the people who were killed.'"
>
> (Nussbaum, 1995, p. 68)

Nussbaum draws from this exchange a lesson against complacency, against the idea that somehow the numbers "buy off" the deaths and make them morally inconsequential. Because Sissy's remarks are apt no matter how few the number of deaths, other readers might draw a stronger lesson—that even one death is too many, and that we therefore should never deliberately pursue policies that put people at risk for the sake of some larger, but non-vital benefit. Nussbaum herself won't go this far, since she thinks "we certainly should be ready to accept a relatively low risk of death or disease to attain considerable social gains"

(Nussbaum, 1995, p. 69). She makes this more cautious interpretation of Dickens because she is aware of the theoretical and practical problems with believing that every life is of infinite value.[4] This is an understanding of moral complexity that she brings to her reading of the book, and without it, her morality is likely to be led astray by the novel. This is because of the strength of Dickens' art, not because of any defect in it. If Sissy had replied to M'Choakumchild with a disquisition on risk–benefit analysis, she would no longer be believable as a character whose voice carries rhetorical and emotional force. And if Dickens had written *Hard Times* to ensure that it fairly portrayed all of the issues involved in making utilitarian tradeoffs, it would have ended up a Socratic dialogue rather than a novel.

All of the above is to emphasize what Nussbaum acknowledges but other commentators sometimes glide over: that stories by themselves, no matter how well written, are not reliable moral guides.[5] They may serve to bring to the table a moral point of view, a set of experiences, or a perspective that otherwise might have been overlooked, and this is a valuable role. But we should not exaggerate the value of reading stories. Stories are not the only route to the discovery of alternative viewpoints, and so are not indispensable for ethical reflection. And perspectives when offered through a story are not thereby privileged moral knowledge. They are claims like any other, which must be evaluated by extra-narrative means.

Bridging the Gap

Another kind of epistemic claim made on behalf of narrative is that it bridges the gap between abstract ethical principles and the concrete circumstances of real cases; that with it, we can remedy the problem of interpretation plaguing abstract principles.

As Hunter puts it, "Narrative negotiates the application of general truths about human experience to the individual case" (Hunter, 1995, p. 1791). Leder contends that narrative understanding is essential because a "'top down' methodology, wherein one commences with high-level theory, can obscure the rich complexity of cases." Rather than whether to tell the patient the truth about his cancer, we need to know how much truth to tell, what counts as the "truth," what the patient will hear when we tell the truth, etc. "A hermeneutic approach, oriented toward the close reading of narratives, may better note the significance of such elements imperceptible from the heights of ethical theory" (Leder, 1984, p. 251).

How? What is the medium through which narrative makes this connection? The one most frequently invoked is "interpretation." But what is "interpretation," how is it distinct from appeals to principled moral commitment, and how could it tie principles to particulars? A few examples will illustrate the significance of these questions.

Drew Leder describes a mother deciding whether to authorize surgery for a severely deformed newborn, and asserts that the case "provokes broad *interpretive* conflicts. . . Is this newborn a full-fledged person in danger of being subjected to the cruelest form of discrimination. . . a dying child whose suffering may be needlessly prolonged. . . not a 'person' at all?" (Leder, 1984, pp. 243–244; my emphasis).

How is it useful or illuminating to say that these disagreements are about matters of "interpretation" rather than about the substance and relevance of ethical principles? How will we decide among these alternatives if not by critically examining our principled commitments regarding respecting persons, having a right to life, avoiding discrimination, and so on? And if interpretation is a form of reflection to be employed in addition to, rather than instead of, principled reasoning, what is it that distinguishes "interpretive" from "principled" modes of critical ethical judgment?

As if to clarify this distinguishing feature, Leder remarks that hermeneutics (understood here as the discipline of interpretation) is a "communal dialogue which progresses through revelatory give and take" (Leder, 1984, p. 254). In a similar direction, Rita Charon asserts than one "locates the authority for judging a conclusion's rightness of fit [with the narrative] on its acceptability to others doing similar work" (Charon, 1994, p. 273).

Not very helpful. *Any* social system of reasoned reflection involves a "communal dialogue" of "give and take," including those deliberately rooted in principle. Charon's Kuhnian account gets us no further: it doesn't distinguish ethics, from science, from anthropology, from literary criticism, because it glides over the question of what features govern "acceptability."

The failure to provide any more precise account of the nature and role of "interpretation" is a symptom of the tendency to wave it and "narrative" as banners that fly over everything bright and beautiful being ignored by those crude and insensitive principles. In standard bioethics discussions of surrogate motherhood, for example, Leder claims that "so much remains unconsidered. . . market pressures and alienating labor-options that may lead women to become surrogate mothers; the fetishism of commodities described by Marx, and how this infiltrates our treatment of human beings; the way gender roles as conceived of within our society shape our notions of 'motherhood'" (Leder, 1984, p. 253). (Notice, incidentally, that these are all concerns motivated by worry over the genuineness of the surrogate mother's "autonomy," and hence they all arise out of allegiance to a moral principle.) Now if all these different inquiries involve the use of "interpretation," then the term has come to apply to virtually any account whatsoever, framed within any set of methods. Conceived so globally, "interpretation" can't be a construct useful for demarcating any distinctive way of understanding and resolving ethical problems.

Can we get a better fix on the relevant features of "interpretation"? Advocates of narrative ethics need to, because some of the characteristics that one would naively attribute to "interpretation" belie the claim that a narrative ("interpretive") ethics avoids the reliance upon abstractions that is the chief sin of "principlism." In one core sense of the word, to "interpret" a set of events is to assign it a meaning that places those events within some larger framework. That framework will of necessity be composed of more general and abstract commitments and beliefs. An example comes from Charles Radey's discussion of a man facing death in an ICU.

> "One way of considering our ICU case is to see this man in terms of myth. Surely he is coming to grips with death, its meaning in his life, and the possibilities of rebirth... The mythical realm opens, requiring courage and inviting discovery. Familiarity with the grand stories and myths of the ages prepares the practitioner as well as the patient for terminal-care decisions."
>
> (Radey, 1992, p. 42)

Unfortunately, Radey never gets any more specific than this, but we know the sort of "myths" and metaphors he's probably referring to. Our culture offers us images of Death as the grim reaper, or the merciful angel delivering us from the mortal coil, or the endless sleep, or the door to eternity, and so on. Any of these metaphors might shape in some way the patient's or practitioner's response to impending death. But the guidance they offer for specific choices and responses is, if anything, even more amorphous and abstract that the most general ethical principle. How could "interpretation" provide the missing link between abstract ethical principle and concrete specifics if interpretation itself is inherently an act of abstraction?

Another difficulty with employing "interpretation" as a tool for concretizing ethical principles gets uncovered when we ask when it is that we most feel the need to supply interpretations. One answer is that we are driven to interpretation when situations present us with recalcitrant ambiguities and apparent contradictions. Interpretations are attempts to resolve or account for these in some coherent way; the more complex the circumstances, and the better our imaginations and other interpretive resources, the greater the variety of alternative interpretations. If the situation is one that presents us with an ethical problem, a central ethical question will then become, "Which interpretation should we act on?" It remains a mystery how this question is to be answered through the medium of interpretation itself. Interpretation has supplied the alternatives; it has not provided any resolution. If interpretations are to help resolve choices, it will be because they supply reasons for preferring one alternative over another. And supplying reasons is to appeal to abstractions and generalizations of some magnitude.

Indeed, the richer and more interpretable the story, the less the resolution offered for the ethical questions raised within it. It's instructive here to compare Richard Selzer's "Mercy" with Timothy Quill's "Death and Dignity" (the story of "Diane"). "Mercy" invites competing interpretations of facts and motives at every turn. This is what makes it a pleasing work of art; but it is also what leaves the reader at sea with respect to any final judgment whether the physician acted rightly in the story by not giving the final, fatal dose, let alone with respect to any more general judgment about the ethics of assisted suicide and euthanasia. By contrast, Quill's story of Diane is a set-piece constructed deliberately at every turn to persuade the reader that Quill acted ethically, and to make the case for assisted suicide as an option for patients. But to accomplish this, Quill has to submerge any opportunities for the reader to supply alternative interpretations of events. So, for example, he tells us that it was "clear that preoccupation with her fear of a lingering death would interfere with Diane's getting the most out of the time she had left" (Quill, 1991, p. 693). We don't get to hear the conversations that led Quill to that conclusion, and so we're presented with no opportunity to provide our own, perhaps very different, interpretation of their meaning.

The point is not to attribute any dishonesty to Quill, but to emphasize a common feature of interpretation: it may as often complicate choice as clarify or resolve it. Not that complicating choice is a bad thing, or useless as an element in ethical deliberation. We should fully appreciate when genuine complexity faces us, and if alternative interpretations can expose that complexity, then that is an honorable role for interpretive skill, which I will discuss more fully shortly. Interpretation just can't play the mediator between principles and particulars, where the gap looms just a large as before narrative stepped up to the plate.

This point has implications for the plausibility of the idea that casuistry (discussed in the previous chapter) provides the normative method of choice for narrative, a notion advanced by Kathryn Montgomery Hunter, among others (Hunter, 1995 and 1997). It has always struck me that what are usually offered as paradigm cases (in both classical and contemporary casuistry) are incredibly thin "narratives." And how could it be otherwise? Thicken them up and you get ethics gumbo. Their status as paradigm cases (which must by definition evoke an unambiguous moral response) would evaporate and their comparison with problematic cases become hopelessly complicated. To function as moral paradigms, they must be archetypes immune to interpretation, not narratives richly interpretable.

Perhaps we need Joanne Trautmann Banks' reminder that literary works are not arguments. She contrasts George Bernard Shaw's preface to his play *The Doctor's Dilemma* with the play itself:

> "When he writes polemical prose, Shaw argues easily, logically, and from an unshakeable moral perspective. But when he takes ethics into the personal realm of drama, he cannot manage equally clear conclusions. So the play, as distinct from the preface, reverberates with moral ambiguity."
>
> (Banks, 1995, p. 1373)

This suggests that narratives must play a role distinctly different than ethical argument or reasoning. We will want to see what that role is, and whether and how the two might complement one another. Before doing so, we should consider one version of the idea that narratives are implicit arguments.

Narrative Rationality

Some have suggested that any ongoing narrative, and especially the "narrative" of an individual life, carries with it an internal rationality that elevates one choice over another as the right or best one. Alasdair MacIntyre points out that we cannot understand any individual human action without placing it within a history of some sort: "in successfully identifying and understanding what someone else is doing we always move towards placing a particular episode in the context of a set of narrative histories. . . action itself has a basically historical character" (MacIntyre, 1984, pp. 211–212).

It is not just other people's lives that we understand properly as stories, but our own. "Man is in his actions and practice, as well as in his fictions, essentially a story-telling animal. . . I can only answer the question 'What am I to do' if I can answer the prior question 'Of what story or stories do I find myself a part?' (MacIntyre, 1984, p. 216). He means to refer here to more than the fact that in order to comprehend the consequences of my choices, I must understand how others are likely to respond to them, where their responses will be shaped by historically conditioned expectations and conventions. Rather, the story of my life demands a narrative coherence that makes one choice more intelligible than another. "In what does the unity of an individual life consist? The answer is that its unity is the unity of a narrative embodied in a single life. . . To ask 'What is the good for me?' is to ask how best I might live out that unity and bring it to completion" (MacIntyre, 1984, p. 218).

This view is carried over into medical ethics by proponents of narrative who assert that we can best gauge the ethics of choices made by or for patients by attending to how those choices fit into the fabric of the patient's story. Writing about the ethics of decisions for incompetent elderly persons, Howard Brody argues "that among those things to be considered are the elements of the life narrative that is drawing to a close, and which sorts of endings make the most sense within the context of that narrative" (Brody 1987, p. 164; emphasis in the original).

The fundamental fallacy in these views is the inference from the claim that my life is best *described* by a narrative to the normative claim that my life choices are best judged by their coherence within my life narrative. My history (my story so far) will shape what I do no matter what I do. And no matter what I do it will be intelligible within "the" narrative of my life. MacIntyre and others reify "my narrative" as if it were a kind of script being followed. Hence, the phrase "the narratives we live out." Unless we assume that our stories are being written by someone else (God, or the Fates), we don't live out a narrative, we create one by living a life. Of course, the narrative we create is a unity, as MacIntyre says. It is the story of our life. But the narrative of the individual life (of the single choosing agent) is necessarily a unity. It may end up a tragic narrative, or a fool's narrative, or a noble narrative. They will all equally be narrative unities. As John Christman puts it, "If one grants that the individual in question is a conscious reflecting interpreter of her own experiences, then the thematic unity [of a narrative] will be achieved whenever the interpreting subject can make minimal sense of her experiences, where 'sense' is not specified in advance. The further insistence that the experiences of which she is a subject be *narrative* in form adds nothing to the analysis" (Christman, 1998, p. 10).

So the question of how best to live out "that" unity is not answered by the notion of narrative unity. It's answered by appeal to extra-narrative ideals that elevate some kinds of narratives over others. Howard Brody, for example, incorporates ideals of moral integrity and human relationship into his conception of narrative ethics: "When we have a momentous decision to make, we often ask ourselves how that decision would fit within our unfolding life story. Would it cohere in a meaningful and authentic way as the sort of action that the principal character of this narrative would be likely to perform?" (Brody, 1992, p. 249). Elsewhere, he suggests that a coherent life story is one in which my actions "appear reasonable and responsible" rather than "whimsical and aberrant" and is "a story of a person who cares what his close associates think of him" (Brody, 1994, p. 210). Well, that's one kind of story, and it could be a pretty dull one from the sound of it. The lives of an expedient scoundrel or a moral chameleon or a flinty loner would equally well be narratives, and *as narratives* they could be equally coherent (and maybe more interesting). They may not be equally worthy *as lives*, but if so it is because we are judging them against conceptions of the best way to live, not conceptions of the best way to write or tell a story.

When advocates of narrative ethics forget this, their ethics is presumed rather than argued for. Arthur Frank's *The Wounded Storyteller: Body, Illness and Ethics* is a case in point. In the book, Frank wants to point out that those who are sick have ethical choices to make regarding how they are going to continue their lives as persons. They may choose between types of body-selves, whether the disciplined body, the dominating body, the mirroring body, or the communicative body, each of which reflect various combinations of attitudes toward one's illness, one's own body, other persons, and so on. And these choices will shape the kind of story one makes out of the illness experience: it might be a restitution narrative, a chaos narrative, or a quest narrative.

Although at times Frank's postmodern allegiances might suggest otherwise,[6] he wants these to be more than descriptive categories in a sociology of illness: hence the "ethics" in his title. Thus, the body types are "types of ethical choices" (Frank, 1997, p. 37), and these choices should be gauged against certain standards for a "good" story. "Stories have to <u>repair</u> the damage that illness has done" (Frank, 1997, p. 53; his emphasis). "The good story refuses denial" and through it "the ill person rises to the occasion" (Frank, 1997, p. 63). "The good story ends in wonder" at the ability to reclaim a self and an ongoing narrative out of the narrative wreckage dealt by illness (Frank, 1997, p. 68). And "good" stories are testimonies, told not just to oneself but to others who may then draw power from them (Frank, 1997, Chapter 7). Given these standards, it is not surprising that Frank endorses the communicative body creating a quest narrative as the ethical ideal for the ill person.

But these ethical standards are not derived from or warranted by any of the narrative types themselves. They are brought to the narratives, as ideals, precepts, or goals extrinsic to narrative, but by which the narratives are to be judged and compared. Narratives that don't meet these standards will be nonetheless narratives. Even the chaos narrative will be a narrative, the story of a life for whom the world no longer makes sense. As extrinsic ideals, these standards need to be defended, but Frank does very little in this direction beyond barely articulating them. To be resigned to loss, to rail at a capricious God, to seek escape (or honor the old self that is lost) through suicide, rather than to seek transformation through suffering, are all on Frank's account less honorable responses to illness. And maybe they are. But supporting this ethic requires reasons that go beyond inspiring stories of illness like those of Gilda Radner, Stuart Alsop, Norman Cousins, or Robert Murphy, which are no more coherent illness narratives than those with less heroic ambitions.

None of the above denies that my life's narrative unity demands some coherence with my history of values, relation-ships, and choices. But since that coherence can be achieved through indefinitely many routes, the "demand" of narrative coherence becomes so easily met as to lose virtually all of its pre-scriptive force. Margaret Urban Walker agrees that in deciding what to do, an individual will feel the need to take account of his or her individual, historically shaped hierarchies of ideals and values. But in so taking account, the person is engaged in what she calls "moral self-definition"—not merely living out an iden-tity, but creating one. One's particular judgments are "undertak-ings." They are not contracts binding on some future self, because my future self retains the capacity for moral self-definition and redefinition. "Particulars presumed to apply on the basis of past concerns and commitments may be revoked or revised, as well as renewed. . . To affirm a moral position on the basis of weighting certain particulars is either. . . to sustain an extant moral course or to chart. . . a new one" (Walker, 1987, p. 179). The need for moral self-definition, like the need for narrative coherence, leaves open questions about which past concerns and commitments will be revoked, how they may be revised, and how past choices will be interpreted. My choices must be made only *within* an historical, narrative context; they are not made by it.

Take as an example the sort of situation that Howard Brody suggests would be best understood by attending to narrative coherence. An elderly man has completed a durable power of attorney appointing his son as decision-maker, and specifying that he did not want heroic treatments employed if he had a terminal illness. Following a stroke, he remains in the intensive care unit one week later unconscious, with severe, unstable hypotension, managed only with maximum doses of medication. The chances for the return of blood pressure control and for substantial neurological recovery are low, but it is not impossible. His son wants to consider withdrawal of the medication, even given its probably lethal consequences. How would an inquiry into narrative coherence help us evaluate this request? Is there a course of action that would, as a narrative, "make the most sense" as the last chapter in this man's story?

I don't think there is, just because there are an indefinitely large number of next chapters that could make sense. We can start first with the obvious fact that what he meant to commit himself to when he wrote his advance directive is open to multiple interpretations. What did he mean by "heroic" treatment or "terminal" illness? Why did he give his son durable power of attorney—to administer his wishes, or to interpret them? What was most important to him: adherence to his expressed preferences, or fatherly trust in his son's love and judgment? Of course, more details of his story (i.e., more facts) might help rule out some answers as improbable, and lend support to others. But further questions of interpretation will invariably arise at this next level as well. Even if we could settle on a single unambiguous interpretation of his intentions when he signed the advance directive, we would still have the further question of what he would make of those intentions now. Would he reaffirm them; reinterpret them (in what directions?); repudiate them? Finally, to what extent is "his" story a product of his own devising? The last chapter the father would write might well be different than the last chapter his son would write. Each would present a coherent narrative of a life, albeit from a different point of view.

Because there are so many coherent narrative possibilities, the standard of narrative coherence can do little to warrant one line of narrative over another. We will instead turn to other considerations, derived from non-narrative detective work into the facts, from principle and from policy. A principle of respect for autonomy will privilege the father's narrative over the son's equally coherent one. The desirability of preserving the integrity of family decision-making may justify our giving the son the authority to select among competing, but equally coherent, interpretations of his father's wishes; and so on. As I suggested earlier, the pursuit of narrative and interpretive possibilities may appropriately complicate our moral choices, but by itself offers little help in making them.

In the second edition of his *Stories of Sickness* (2003), Brody responds to these arguments by admitting that the norm of narrative coherence requires at the least "that we *want* our lives to be coherent as narrative." But this won't be enough to evaluate alternative narratives when there are so many possibilities open, all of which would be equally narratives. Brody feels compelled, accordingly, to add something beyond this minimal norm. Following Walker, the additional moral constraint is that we should want to be seen as "reliable," so that "our associates. . . can reasonably predict how we will behave in a wide variety of circumstances" (Brody, 2003. p. 219). This is a substantive norm, and drawing on it concedes my point. If I am unpredictable, it doesn't mean that there is no story to be told about my life and behavior. It may not be the most desirable life from the point of view of those relying on me, but there's a story to be told about it, both by others and by me. Even more tellingly, if we were to grant that reliability is the norm by which narrative coherence should be judged, it would surely not be the only norm to which we were committed, or even the most important. I would have decisions to make about when my life should be reliable (viz. "coherent") and when coherence should take a back seat to my other values. When the meaning of "narrative coherence" is specified by reference to a non-narrative norm, we can make judgments about which stories are the more coherent alright; but the decision about when to be coherent moves out of the realm of narrative evaluation.

One more point. When we consider the usefulness of narratives as a tool for warranting particular moral choices concerning patients, we should not confuse the idea of narrative coherence with inferences from generalizations about human nature. Take as an example of such confusion Mark W. Waymack's claim that regarding particular patients, "narrative ethics offers the story as the guide to decision making" (Waymack, 1996, p. 2). He illustrates this claim with the situation of an elderly, demented, and gravely ill woman without family or friends, where decisions must be made whether to admit her to the intensive care unit to attempt to treat her advancing pneumonia:

"If, however, we can 'learn' the patient's story, we will thereby learn what drives the biography. . . And as we hear the preceding chapters, it becomes easier to discern how the next chapter should be written. Think how our decision making might swing in the case of Mrs. A if we knew, for example, that she had in her earlier old age been a sustaining volunteer for a hospice organization. . . Such a narrative could greatly contribute to our construction of plot lines for the final chapters of her life that would be consistent with the earlier chapters of her personal narrative."

(Waymack, 1996, p. 2)

Are we supposed to think that someone who had been a hospice volunteer earlier in her life would be a person who abhorred aggressive treatment at the end of life, and who would now tell us to let her die in peace, if only she could speak? But this is a presumption based on a simple (and crudely stereotypical) generalization about those who volunteer in hospices. There is nothing remotely "personal" about it, and in its inattention to the texture of Mrs. A's life, character, or motives, it is the antithesis of narrative. It may indeed be the best evidence we have. But if it warrants any decisions about how to care for Mrs. A, it won't be due to its place in any narrative.

A Role for Narrative: Telling More Stories

I want now to pick up a thread dropped earlier—that narratives may provide a medium through which we come to a more complex understanding of the ethical situation before us. This is a virtue of narratives that makes good use of an important contrast with principles and rules. Narratives are particularizing, where principles are abstracting. It is through abstraction that principles become useful as reasons supporting a point of view, because in generalizing they draw on a range of moral attitudes across a variety of particular circumstances. An appeal to respect for autonomy becomes a reason to get John's informed consent for a treatment because it points (however vaguely) to other moral commitments we have regarding autonomy, including commitments to persons in circumstances quite different than John's. Since narratives move away from abstraction, they tend to be less useful as reasons-for-conclusions, but more useful in highlighting ethically relevant particulars that would otherwise have been overlooked in a rush to principles. An account of the details of conversation between John and his physician, for example, might lead us at various points to wonder how well he understood his choices. Although a narrative account wouldn't answer these questions, without its level of detail and context they wouldn't have arisen at all.

I think there are two ways in which narrative can be used appropriately to enrich the moral picture, and they both involve our capacity to tell stories. One is an aid to our moral investigation, the other an aid to our moral imagination.

Getting All the Stories

Regardless of their epistemological bent, everyone in medical ethics will agree that one needs to "get the whole story" to make an informed judgment about the moral choices posed by particular situations. This is true even of those who believe that moral theory and principles are the key moral ingredients in moral deliberation.

But how does one "get the whole story"? As narrativists remind us, the facts of a case are never all collected together in a box, ready to hand for us to sort through as we will. They are always *presented* to us in some form or another—as a case report, someone's verbal description, a set of progress notes, or even in our own mental rehearsal of what we think we know. This presentation is always partial, in the several senses of that word. It never contains within it all of the facts, but only some selection of them; and it selects and orders those facts in certain ways rather than in others, ways that imply differences in relevance, importance, causation, and motivation. Thus, "the" facts are always represented to us as narratives (in some broad, and not necessarily literary, sense of that term). As Tod Chambers famously points out, the case narrative may well be "framed in ways that conceal as well as reveal other ways of seeing" (Chambers, 1996, p. 32). Becoming more richly aware of the facts and perspectives that are concealed in presented narratives requires that one be able to tell alternative versions of the story, which point to questions of fact that remain to be answered.

Take as an example a case used by Hilde Lindemann Nelson to illustrate the importance of what she calls "counterstories" (Nelson, 1997b), referencing a discussion of a case by Fleck and Angell:

"The patient, Carlos R, was a twenty-one-year-old Hispanic male who had suffered gunshot wounds to the abdomen in gang violence. He was uninsured. His stay in the hospital was somewhat shorter than might have been expected, but otherwise unremarkable. It was felt that he could safely complete his recovery at home. Carlos admitted to his attending physician that he was HIV-positive, which was confirmed.

At discharge the attending physician recommended a daily home nursing visit for wound care. However, Medicaid would not fund this nursing visit because a caregiver lived in the home who could adequately provide this care, namely, the patient's twenty-two-year-old sister Consuela, who in fact was willing to accept this burden. Their mother had died almost ten years ago, and Consuela had been a mother to Carlos and their younger sister since then. Carlos had no objection to Consuela's providing this care, but he insisted absolutely that she was not to know his HIV status. He had always been on good terms with Consuela, but she did not know he was actively homosexual. His greatest fear, though, was that his father would learn of his homosexual orientation, which is generally looked upon with great disdain by Hispanics.

Would Carlos's physician be morally justified in breaching patient confidentiality on the grounds that he had a "duty to warn"?"

(Fleck and Angell, 1991, p. 39)

Commenting on the case, Leonard Fleck analyzes its issues in terms of well-accepted, standard criteria for a "duty to warn." There must be "(1) an imminent threat of serious and irreversible harm, (2) no alternative to averting that threat other than this breach of confidentiality, and (3) proportionality between the harm averted by this breach of confidentiality and the harm associated with such a breach" (Fleck and Angell, 1991, p. 39). After discussing the low likelihood that Consuela would become HIV-infected, the alternative of her using universal precautions, and the real social and other harms that Carlos might suffer if his HIV status and his homosexuality are disclosed, Fleck concludes that these criteria are not satisfied and so the physician has no duty to warn Consuela.

Given the way the story is written, Fleck's analysis makes good sense. But notice that this story—like all stories—is written from a particular point of view, and with an emphasis on certain features of the situation to the exclusion of others. This is the story as it might be written by the physician. There is an emphasis on the medical aspects of the problem (Carlos' need for home care; the risks of HIV transmission), and the social aspects are recounted from the point of view of the protagonist the physician has spoken with and has professional loyalties to.

Drawing on work by Margaret Urban Walker (Walker, 1993), Nelson points out that the story leaves out other points of view and characters whose further narrative development might suggest additional facts of moral relevance. For example, the story that Carlos tells about Consuela suggests someone who has selflessly taken on responsibility for caring for her family: she "has been a mother to Carlos and their younger sister" since their mother died. To call her a "mother" is to assign her to a role that carries implicit moral duties, in particular the duty to care for her "children" even at some sacrifice of her own interests. Maybe this is really the heart of Consuela's story. But one can imagine at least that she might tell it differently. Perhaps she would tell a story of oppression, Nelson suggests, that exposes how her traditional family and the social system around it have unfairly treated her, thwarting her every attempt to break free into a life she can call her own.

By articulating these alternative story possibilities, we may reveal additional features of the situation that will be relevant to our moral understanding of it. This relevance can be of two kinds. In the first instance, alternative narratives might suggest further factual questions that require some investigation because they are relevant to the terms of our initial moral analysis. Consuela's "counterstory," for example, suggests that she may harbor a level of resentment and suspicion that would make it unlikely that she would be satisfied with a vague and general rationale for her use of universal precautions. If further investigation confirmed that this was indeed the case, this is an additional fact that might alter the moral conclusion of Fleck's analysis, because it undermines the possibility that there is a viable alternative to disclosure that will secure the home care services that Carlos needs. Even though its conclusion may change, the terms of that analysis remain unchanged.

Expanding What's at Stake

Alternative narratives have another use that is less mundane in its implications. They may suggest that there are additional moral considerations or principles at stake that were previously unrecognized; they may change the terms of the moral analysis by expanding our moral imaginations. Again, Consuela's imagined counterstory suggests an example of this. If all her life she has chafed under systematic exploitation and injustice, then we may wonder whether our securing her services for Carlos by withholding information from her just takes advantage of and perpetuates her exploitation. Or we might think that under the circumstances Carlos owes her a special duty of disclosure, as a form of restitution for the advantages he's taken and enjoyed. Under the previous terms of the moral analysis, the only pertinent question regarding Consuela was whether non-disclosure threatened her with some significant risk of harm. The expanded story indicates we should also ask whether nondisclosure *wrongs* her by violating a duty we or Carlos owe to her. As Walker puts it, "Carlos's and Consuela's stories, in social perspective, draw other general concerns of self and mutual respect, filial obligation, gratitude, and trust into the picture" (Walker 1993, p. 36).

Take as another example an article sometimes taken to exemplify the narrative approach to an ethical problem. In the article, William F. May approaches the famous case of Dax Cowart not by setting up an argument from ethical principles regarding autonomy and the justification of paternalism (although he gets to these in the end), but by systematically describing, in horrific and vivid detail, the catastrophe of pain, loss, and self-loathing resulting from severe burns like Dax's. Although May's account is more a general phenomenology of the burn victim's experience than a narrative, it serves a similar purpose, by portraying the felt inner experience of someone like Dax. The effect of May's account is to portray the degree to which a patient like Dax faces not just a choice between life and death, or a choice between quality and quantity of life, but an existential choice whether to leap into an unknown future where a new identify might perhaps be found:

> "Thrown out into a no-man's-land, without much resource from his or her former life, cut off from former goals, old skills suddenly irrelevant, aspirations utterly unattainable, old identities and enthusiasms on the ash heap, the old persona unwearable, and the familiar rhythms and tempo of life faltering, such an individual faces far more than a quandary to be solved. In an unheroic age, the survivor must unexpectedly push out into the unknown, where each day is an agony, without a new identity in place."
>
> (May, 1989, pp. 146–147)

The ethical point is not to displace the ethical analysis that focuses on whether to honor Dax's persistent refusals of life-saving treatment, the focus of another essay in the same volume by James Childress and Courtney Campbell. It is rather, as Paul Lauritzen has it, that "the conventional analysis of such cases in bioethics, the sort of analysis offered by Childress and Campbell that pits paternalism against autonomy, is incomplete" (Lauritzen, 1996, p. 11). May's vivid portrayal of the patient's experience reminds us of at least two other sorts of ethical questions. One is the ethical question facing the patient: whether to be the sort of "hero" May says the choice to go on requires, or whether to give up in despair at the enormity of the wreckage that remains of one's life. The other is a related question that faces Dax's caregivers and our social system: whether we have a duty to provide the sorts of resources, many of them non-medical and non-technical, that may make the heroic choice a bit less daunting. The ethical question that concerns Childress and

Campbell is not an unimportant one; it is, after all, the question that Dax's refusal of treatment poses most immediately to his caregivers, from the point of view of their experience of the moral conflict that this refusal creates for them. May's strategy is to change the perspective from which the situation is viewed, and as with Consuela's story, its effect is to introduce ethical dimensions that were otherwise hidden from view.

There are two remaining points to be made about the uses of narrative imagination to "tell the whole story." The first is that narrative imagination can be useful whether the new or expanded stories that get told turn out to be true or not. Consuela's real story may be nothing like Nelson's portrayal of oppression, but the imaginative portrayal makes it apparent why it may be important for us to find out more about Consuela's real story, and identifies at least some of the questions about it we will want to answer. May doesn't much bother to confirm the extent to which Dax's particular experience of his burns and their psychic and spiritual aftermath was like May's general portrayal. Doesn't matter: May's claim that there are important ethical questions in these cases other than the choice between autonomy and paternalism remains.

The second point expands one made earlier: narrative detail increases ethical complexity, but is poorly suited by itself for supporting one choice over another. That will require non-narrative resources. Consuela's story of oppression raises the possibility that Carlos owes her a duty of disclosure. But whether we should believe that he in fact has such a duty, or that it is strong enough to override his caregivers' duty of confidentiality, are questions that require us to resort to the language of principles, placing such questions within a larger framework of moral commitments.

This is not to say that narratives cannot help inform some uses of principles. One such role draws on Mill's famous dictum regarding how one could make a reasoned comparison of two pleasures to decide which one was the higher:

> "Of two pleasures, if there be one to which all or almost all who have experience of both give a decided preference, irrespective of any feeling of moral obligation to prefer it, that is the more desirable pleasure."
>
> (Mill, 1957, p. 12)

Mill's point is that there is no way to know whether poetry is a higher pleasure than push-pin except through having experienced both pleasures. The judgment of those who have put themselves in a position to know is the only warrant available for any claim that one is better than another.

In a similar vein, we might say that there is no way to know whether violating our duty to Consuela threatens a greater harm than violating our duty to Carlos except by having experience of both of these harms. But how is this possible? Unlike the pleasures of push-pin and poetry, we can't put ourselves in the position of having direct acquaintance with the experiences of either Carlos or Consuela, let alone each of them in turn. Their respective stories, however, may offer us sources of insightful appreciation of the nature and magnitudes of the harms each may suffer if his or her moral claims are not honored. If, after eliciting these stories and discussing our understandings of them, we come to agreement about the relative magnitudes of harm each portrays, then the stories would have helped to warrant that comparative moral judgment. This suggests that narratives may be a tool we can use to justify the balancing judgments the use of principles requires, but for which principles themselves can provide no justification.

Two cautions will limit this use of narratives to warrant balancing judgments. The first, of course, concerns the need to develop credible stories for valid comparisons. We will need to make sure that the stories of all the relevant parties are brought into play (e.g., including Carlos' and Consuela's father). We will need to assess the stories for their consistency with other information we have. We will need to agree that the stories are stylistically comparable (e.g., that one doesn't use dramatic devices to unfairly elevate the emotional impact of its portrayal). We will need to arrive at agreement about the interpretation of the events and characters portrayed, and so on. At each of these points, there is likely to be contention, and the disagreements may turn out to be intractable.

The other caution points out that evaluation of the weight of competing duties or principles has to do with more than the harms that might befall those involved (unless, perhaps, we are act utilitarians). Even if we can agree, on the basis of their respective stories, that Consuela will suffer the greater harm from having her claims overridden, it may still be the case that our duty to Carlos is the greater one. Perhaps the claim for a duty to Consuela is less well supported by appeals to other principles or judgments in reflective equilibrium. Perhaps the duty to Carlos has deeper connections to other important social institutions, like the doctor–patient relationship, so that its violation would have more significant reverberations for our common life. Balancing any competing duties to Carlos and Consuela will require our evaluation and judgment regarding these sorts of dimensions as well, where narrative is not as apt a tool. Evaluating duties for their inferential connections to other duties and principles or for their social embeddedness requires a level of abstraction and generality and modes of justification that are at odds with the particularity of narratives.

Recourse to narratives, then, can help us make some small progress in addressing the balancing problem, but we will need to be wary of its limitations.

Conclusion

So how can narrative thinking aid us in warranting out moral judgments? I've identified a few modest but significant ways. Stories can expand our understanding of other people and perhaps ourselves, so that our ethical judgments become better informed. They may awaken moral sensibilities so that we more keenly feel the wrongfulness of circumstances we had become hardened or blind to. The imperative to "get the whole story," and the interpretive skills that help to do so, can help uncover ethically relevant complexities. And narratives may be one means for comparing some of the moral consequences of alternative courses of action.

What remains untenable is the idea that narrative provides a mode of ethical justification that is independent from or superior to appeals to moral principles. Neither interpretation nor narrative coherence offers the tools needed for choosing from among all the interpretive and narrative possibilities.

Notes

1. This chapter is based on my previous article "Perplexed by Narrative Ethics" (Tomlinson, 1997).

2. Hilde Lindemann Nelson, remarking on Richard Rorty's claim that literary critics make the best moral advisors because they have (at least vicariously) been around, points out that "whether literary critics are competent moral advisors has less to do with where they have been than with how they behaved when they got there" (Nelson, 2001, p. 51).

3. Here I am borrowing not quite all of the ways to use stories that Hilde Nelson has described. We can read them, compare them, analyze them, invoke them, and tell them (Nelson 1997a, pp. x–xii) She has recently added that we can "uncover" them, a category I will make use of later (Nelson, unpublished manuscript).

4. See Fleck (1990) for a discussion of these problems in the health care context.

5. "[M]y view does not urge a naive uncritical reliance on the literary work. I have insisted that the conclusions we are apt to draw on the basis of our literary experience need the continued scrutiny of moral and political thought, of our own moral and political intuitions, and of the judgments of others" (Nussbaum, 1995, p. 76).

6. See Arras (1997) for a critical discussion of the subjectivism that Arras thinks derives from Frank's postmodern stance.

Bibliography

Arras, John D. 1997. "Nice Story, But So What?" In *Stories and Their Limits*, ed. Hilde Nelson. New York: Routledge, pp. 65–88.

Banks, Joanne Trautmann. 1995. "Literature." *Encyclopedia of Bioethics*, ed. Warren Thomas Reich. New York: Simon and Schuster, pp. 1369–1376.

Brody, Howard. 1987. *Stories of Sickness*. New Haven: Yale University Press.

Brody, Howard. 1992. *The Healer's Power*. New Haven: Yale University Press.

Brody, Howard. 1994. "The Four Principles and Narrative Ethics." In *Principles of Health Care Ethics*, ed. R. Gillon. London: John Wiley and Sons, pp. 207–215.

Brody, Howard. 2003. *Stories of Sickness*, 2nd ed. Cambridge: Oxford University Press.

Burrell, David and Hauerwas, Stanley. 1977. "From System to Story: An Alternative Pattern for Rationality in Ethics." In *Knowledge, Value, and Belief*, ed. H. Tristram Engelhardt, Jr. and Daniel Callahan. Hastings-on-Hudson, NY: Hastings Center, pp. 111–152.

Chambers, Tod. 1996. "From the Ethicist's Point of View: The Literary Nature of Ethical Inquiry." *Hastings Center Report* 26(1): 25–33.

Charon, Rita. 1994. "Narrative Contributions to Medical Ethics: Recognition, Formulation, Interpretation, and Validation in the Practice of the Ethicist." In Edwin R. Dubose, Ronald P. Hamel, and Laurence J. O'Connell, eds., *A Matter of Principles? Ferment in U.S.*

Bioethics. Valley Forge, PA: Trinity Press International, pp. 260–283.

Childress, James F. and Courtney C. Campbell. 1989. "'Who Is a Doctor to Decide Whether a Person Lives or Dies?' Reflections on Dax's Case." In *Dax's Case: Essays in Medical Ethics and Human Meaning*, ed. Lonnie D. Kliever. Dallas: Southern Methodist University Press, pp. 23–41.

Christman, John. 1998. "Narrative Unity as a Condition of Personhood." Paper presented at the Pacific Division meetings of the American Philosophical Association, Los Angeles, March (Unpublished manuscript).

Diamond, Cora. 1982. "Anything But Argument." *Philosophical Investigations* 5:23–41.

Fleck, Leonard M. 1990. "Pricing Human Life: The Moral Costs of Medical Progress." *The Centennial Review* 34(2):227–253.

Fleck, Leonard and Marcia Angell. 1991. "Please Don't Tell!" *Hastings Center Report*, November–December: 39–40.

Frank, Arthur. 1997. *The Wounded Storyteller: Body, Illness and Ethics.* Chicago: University of Chicago Press.

Hunter, Kathryn Montgomery 1995. "Narrative", *Encyclopedia of Bioethics*, ed. Warren Thomas Reich, vol. 4. New York: Simon & Schuster and Prentice Hall International, pp. 1789–1794.

Hunter, Kathryn Montgomery. 1997. "Aphorisms, Maxims and Old Saws: Narrative Rationality and the Negotiation of Clinical Choice." In *Stories and Their Limits*, ed. Hilde Nelson. New York: Routledge, pp. 215–231.

Lauritzen, Paul. 1996. "Ethics and Experience: The Case of the Curious Response." *Hastings Center Report* 26(1):6–15.

Leder, Drew. 1984. "Toward a Hermeneutical Bioethics." *A Matter of Principles? Ferment in U.S. Bioethics*. Edwin Dubose, Ronald Hamel, and Laurence O'Connell, eds. Valley Forge, PA: Trinity Press International, pp. 240–259.

MacIntyre, Alasdair. 1984. *After Virtue*, 2nd ed. Notre Dame, IN: Notre Dame University Press.

May, William F. 1989. "Dealing with Catastrophe." In *Dax's Case: Essays in Medical Ethics and Human Meaning*, ed. Lonnie D. Kliever. Dallas: Southern Methodist University Press, pp. 131–150.

Mill, John S. 1957. *Utilitarianism*, ed. Oskar Priest. Indianapolis: Bobbs-Merrill.

Nelson, Hilde Lindemann. 1997a. "Introduction: How to Do Things With Stories." In *Stories and Their Limits*, ed. Hilde Nelson. New York: Routledge.

Nelson, Hilde Lindemann. 1997b. "Clinical Counterstories." Paper delivered at the conference *Visions for Ethics and Humanities in a Changing Health Care Environment*, Baltimore, Maryland, Nov. 5–9.

Nelson, Hilde Lindemann. 2001. *Damaged Identities, Narrative Repair*. Ithaca: Cornell University Press.

Nussbaum, Martha C. 1995. *Poetic Justice: The Literary Imagination and Public Life*. Boston: Beacon Press.

Quill, Timothy A. 1991 "Death and Dignity: A Case of Individualized Decision Making." *New England Journal of Medicine* 324:691–694.

Radey, Charles. 1992 "Imagining Ethics: Literature and the Practice of Ethics." *Journal of Clinical Ethics* 3:38–45.

Tomlinson, Tom. 1997. "Perplexed by Narrative Ethics." In *Stories and Their Limits*, ed. Hilde Nelson. New York: Routledge, pp. 123–133.

Selzer, Richard. 1982. "Mercy." *Letters to a Young Doctor*. New York: Simon and Schuster.

Walker, Margaret Urban. 1987. "Moral Particularity." *Metaphilosophy* 18:171–185.

Walker, Margaret Urban. 1993. "Keeping Moral Space Open: New Images of Ethics Consulting." *Hastings Center Report* 23(2):33–40.

Waymack, Mark H. 1996. "Narrative Ethics in the Clinical Setting." *Making the Rounds in Health, Faith and Ethics* 1(15):1–4.

Chapter 6

Feminism, Context, and Care

Feminism as a political cause began well before the turn of the 20th century. As an academic discipline it has been underway at least since the publication of Simone de Beauvoir's *The Second Sex* in 1952. Yet its entry into medical ethics did not really begin until the late 1980s, with the publication of two special issues on medical ethics by the feminist journal *Hypatia*. Since that time, however, feminist scholarship and commentary on ethical issues in health care has grown substantially. Since feminist ethics is often characterized as a distinct method of moral evaluation, it is important to examine its claims in light of my critical discussion of other methods addressed in this book. In what ways is a feminist medical ethic distinctive? If it is distinctive, can it avoid some of the limitations found in other methods, without falling into difficulties of its own?

A major challenge in discussing feminist medical ethics is deciding what one means by a "feminist" ethic. There is a great variety of feminists, many of whom employ methods we've already discussed. In her excellent critical discussion of various forms of feminist ethics, Alison Jaggar lists "feminist Aristotelians,

Humeans, utilitarians, existentialists, and contract theorists as well as 'carers,' 'maternal thinkers,' 'womanists,' and 'spinsters'" among others like "liberals, Marxists and anarchists" (Jaggar, 1991, p. 88).

I have no hope of exploring all of this diversity in what follows, but I do want to capture those aspects of it that are most relevant to the goal of evaluating methods or ways of knowing in medical ethics, and I want to do so in a way that allows me to make critical comparisons between feminist and non-feminist approaches. I will organize the discussion that follows around three ways of conceptualizing feminist ethics. In the first, feminist ethics refers to an objective or *goal* of moral inquiry. In the second, it refers to the use of a distinctive *method* of inquiry. And in the third, it refers to the use of a distinctive *set of normative principles* or commitments. These categories will, I hope, have some heuristic value, but they are not intended to be mutually exclusive. There is no reason a feminist medical ethic couldn't be all three sorts of thing.

A Goal of Inquiry

Feminism, and by extension feminist ethics, is perhaps most commonly thought to be centered around a political or social goal: to identify and to correct those features of the social, cultural, and political environment that contribute to the oppression of women in particular, and of others more generally. Indeed, this is often taken as the core commitment of any feminist ethic, regardless of its other methodological or principled features. As Laura Purdy expresses it:

"At the heart of all feminism...are two simple judgments. First, women are, as a group, worse off than men, because their interests routinely fail to be given equal consideration. Second, that state of affairs is unjust and should be remedied."

(Purdy, 1996, p. 5)[1]

This would seem to set two necessary conditions for any work in medical ethics to be "feminist." Either it must be concerned to show that in the activity under discussion women are disproportionately disadvantaged; or that such a disadvantaging is wrong; or both.

The first condition implies that it will not be enough that discussion is focused on women in general, or even on aspects of health care practices unique to women. We need to avoid the trap of thinking that a discussion in medical ethics that is concerned about a "woman's issue" is thereby feminist.

Nelson and Nelson (1989) invite this confusion, even if they themselves wouldn't fall into it, in an article on surrogate motherhood published in the issue of *Hypatia* that inaugurated feminist medical ethics. The authors critique liberal or contractual models of individual rights and duties that are often taken to support some form of surrogate motherhood. Here they employ standard objections made not only by many feminists, but by other sorts of philosophers as well. At the heart of their argument, however, there is more than a general critique of liberalism. There is the much more specific claim that where one has caused another person to be in need, one has a duty to personally meet those needs, resulting in a responsibility that can't be delegated to someone else. Thus, even in circumstances where the contracting woman's interests as well as those of her child are being well protected, it is a violation of her duty of care to surrender the child to someone else to parent, which is deliberately what happens in surrogate mother arrangements.

Given the conception of "feminist ethics" under discussion, we might ask whether there is anything feminist about this analysis. The principle employed is itself gender-neutral. The sorts of considered judgments the authors use to support it (e.g., the non-contractual duties I acquire when I run over someone with my car) refer to all persons, regardless of gender. The principle applies to both men and women, who are equally vulnerable to violating it. Nelson and Nelson admit, for example, that it implies that sperm donation is ethically dubious as well.

It is really only at the end of their discussion that they make the explicitly feminist connection, when they suggest that their arguments establish that "the assumptions that underlie the practice [of surrogate motherhood] seem to hold an impoverished view of the full significance of women's freedom" (Nelson and Nelson, 1989, p. 94). If their arguments had been directed to such a conclusion, they would indeed have been feminist in their orientation, because at the core would have been the claim that surrogacy unfairly disadvantages or denigrates women. The argument the Nelsons make, however, doesn't show that surrogacy denigrates or diminishes women's freedom, only that women (and men) aren't ethically free to make choices to transfer their parental responsibilities. The objection is that surrogacy invites a parent to do something morally wrong. The fact that in surrogacy that parent is a woman has played no role in the argument. Here I don't mean to dispute their moral criticism of surrogacy.[2] I only mean to dispute the claim that such criticism is feminist, because it is not aimed squarely at establishing some respect in which women are disproportionately disadvantaged.

But there is a more important sort of problem that this first conception of feminist ethics faces, and that arises from the second condition found in Purdy's characterization. Not only must a feminist ethics be concerned to show where women are disadvantaged; it must also be concerned to show that this is wrong. In pursuing this second objective, a feminist agenda encounters the same methodological question we've found with more traditional approaches as well: how to justify the judgment that one moral consideration or objective is weightier than another.

This is as pervasive and perplexing a question for feminist medical ethics as for the other approaches we've been discussing. It arises from the very nature of the feminist project, which is to expose injustice against women. Where such injustice is found, it counts as a relevant and powerful reason against whatever activity or social arrangement creates the injustice. Such enrichment of the ethical discourse is an invaluable role for feminist analysis. But for all that, the sorts of reasons uncovered may not be overriding or decisive considerations, because there may be other morally legitimate and relevant ends that the activity or arrangement fosters. This may be because an activity that subverts justice for women in one respect may serve justice in some other respect. Or it may be because an activity that subverts justice serves some other value besides justice, such as those concerning welfare or individual rights.

Again, the debates over surrogate motherhood can illustrate these possibilities. On the one hand, one might argue that allowing these arrangements unfairly disadvantages the women who participate because they exploit the fact of these women's indoctrination into a sexist ideology, in which childbearing is seen as the ideal—maybe even the only—female role. On the other hand, one might argue that banning surrogate arrangements unfairly disparages the women who would agree to them, by assuming that they are incapable of looking out for themselves. This has the effect of infantilizing these women in a way that wouldn't be tolerated for men. (See Lori Andrews [1988] for some comparison of these arguments.) Perhaps these are both true. Some women would be exploited if surrogacy were permitted, and some women would be infantilized if it were not. But then the problem, for a feminist ethics as for any other, is how to decide which of these injustices is the one most to be avoided.

And there are further balancing judgments to be made as well. So, on the one hand, surrogate arrangements may exploit vulnerable women and so be unjust. But on the other hand, they serve to meet the arguably legitimate needs of infertile women (and their partners) who desire to have children fathered by a particular person. Again, the problem for a feminist ethics, as for any other, is how to determine which of these competing considerations is the more important.

Laura Purdy captures the essential point: "Rectifying gender injustice need not always be our first priority, even if awareness of gender and the difference it makes are always crucial" (Purdy, 1996, p. 5). Both the crucial importance of the awareness of gender and the inadequacy of gender justice as an overarching principle are revealed in another discussion by Nelson and Nelson, this one focusing on the distribution of health care resources.

They take as their guide the core feminist concern with disproportionate burdens: "feminist theory [in the context of distributive justice] . . . accepts the reality of limits [and] is careful to defend women from disproportionate burdens arising from those limits" (Nelson and Nelson, 1996, p. 356). They then give a number of examples of how this concern might be extended in the context under discussion.

One of these addresses cost-containment strategies that reduce high hospital costs by sending patients home as soon as possible, so that the burdens of providing for the patient's further recuperation fall on the family, rather than on the insurer. But, Nelson and Nelson point out, "the family" is a euphemism that in fact is not as gender-neutral as it sounds. Most family caregivers are women, for reasons both of traditional gender roles and economics, and so the burdens of such strategies will fall disproportionately on women. If we didn't already have reasons to question the ethics of such strategies, we do now. Sending patients home "quicker and sicker" is unfair to women as a class of persons.

This is a good example of how a feminist consciousness can help to ferret out morally salient considerations that may otherwise escape notice. A commitment to a principle of distributive justice must be concerned with what the actual distribution is of significant benefits and burdens. If we are insensitive to or ignorant of the effects that gender in fact has on that distribution, then we will be unable to employ the principle in an informed and critical way.

Now that we're convinced that such cost-containment strategies are in this respect unfair to women, then what? We've shown at least that they are *prima facie* wrong, and if there is nothing convincing to be said on their behalf, then they are morally unjustifiable. Perhaps nothing convincing could be said concerning policies that could only be described as sending patients home "quicker and sicker," and so the feminist analysis drives the last nail into that coffin.

In other circumstances, however, the ethical question will be more complicated, and the adequacy of a purely feminist ethics more questionable. Take another argument made by Nelson and Nelson, in which they criticize policies advocated by Daniel Callahan and Norman Daniels that would limit the use of life-prolonging technology in the elderly. As discussed in an earlier chapter, Callahan's and Daniels' position rests on two premises: that justice in health care should aim at distributing an equal opportunity for a normal life span (and the life projects a normal life span makes possible); and that the elderly as a group have already enjoyed this opportunity, and so have no further claims of justice to make against life-prolonging health care resources.

Nelson and Nelson's criticism of this view, borrowed from Nancy Jecker, points out that the elderly have not all equally enjoyed a normal set of life's opportunities, contrary to the assumption made by Callahan and Daniels. Elderly women, in particular, have more often suffered a lifetime of stunted opportunities for the normal range of life projects. Moreover, they add, women's "normal" life span is almost a decade longer than men's, and so a uniform age limit on access to life-prolonging technologies would deprive women of more years of life than it would men. Thus, a policy that on its face appears to disadvantage all of the elderly equally in fact disproportionately disadvantages elderly women by compounding the injustice they have already suffered.

This is an important insight, but what follows from it regarding the justifiability of such a policy? If gender justice is the controlling norm, then the implication is precisely what Nelson and Nelson take it to be: "in deference to women's greater longevity and the need to correct for the sexism that has trammeled their opportunities for self-development, women should be eligible for life-saving interventions for a longer period than are men" (Nelson and Nelson, 1996, p. 362).

But should gender justice be the controlling norm? It is certainly not the only one. There remains the matter of generational justice, which motivated Callahan's concern from the outset. In a environment of limited health care resources for life-prolonging treatment, the elderly, who have already lived a life, will draw resources away from the young, who have not. Which is the greater injustice? To deny the 70-year-old widow treatment that would allow her to live the remainder of her life free of the shackles of traditional marriage and family expectations? Or deny it to the 20-year-old just beginning to pursue his life projects? A feminist focus on gender justice could well obscure other sorts of justice concerns, and in itself cannot warrant a judgment about how these different justice concerns should be prioritized.

This first conception of feminist ethics, then, points up how a feminist consciousness can help us recognize gender-related aspects of policies and practices that warrant our ethical attention. How those feminist concerns are to be weighted, however, will have to be determined within some broader analytical or methodological framework that will still be struggling with the problems of balancing, interpretation, and judgment.

A Method of Inquiry

Many feminist writers, while agreeing that they are concerned with identifying and critiquing disproportionate burdens on women, argue that a feminist ethics also must employ a distinctive method. Perhaps this is most often expressed as a refusal to rely upon abstract principles, insisting instead that we be guided by the richness of specific contexts.

Principles vs. Context

Susan Sherwin, for example, insists that attention to context over abstract principle is a defining feature of a feminist ethic:

> "It is clear that in doing feminist ethics, it is important to be critical of the maleness of mainstream ethical theory, given its tendencies to demand a very high degree of abstractness and to deny the relevance of concrete considerations." (Sherwin, 1989, p. 59)

Even utilitarianism, perhaps the most "context-sensitive" of the standard normative theories, doesn't give context its due. Utilitarianism, Sherwin reminds us, is concerned with impartially calculating the utility values for all of those affected.

But, "in contrast, those engaged in doing feminist or medical ethics often reflect a desire to take account of the details of specific relationships and to give added weight to some particular utility related qualities like caring and responsibility" (Sherwin, 1989, p. 61).

It is important to note that such repudiations of "malestream" ethical traditions and modes of argument are far from uncontroversial within feminist ethics. Alison Jaggar observes that "If claims that Western tradition is masculine mean no more than that it has been constructed primarily by men rather than women, this is neither entirely true. . . nor, in itself, very interesting philosophically," (Jaggar, 1991, p. 89) and asserts that it might often be better for feminists "to appropriate what may have been constructed as the masculine aspects of Western ethics" (Jaggar, 1991, p. 90). Christine Pierce echoes this pragmatic approach. After a critical discussion of the limits of principled and reasoned ethical discourse, she nevertheless concludes that "not all of the laboriously created works of the past are useless for our liberation. Certainly you can destroy the master's house with the master's tools" (Pierce, 1991, 75, putting Audre Lorde's famous dictum on its head).

Even in the feminist medical ethics practiced by Sherwin the relevance of context gets constrained at times by matters of principle. Contrasting standard with feminist medical ethics on the matter of reproductive technologies, for example, Sherwin says that "Feminist theorists. . . are unwilling to allow decisions about such practices. . . to be addressed in isolation from the general pattern constituted by the combined use of these technologies; they resist attempts to decide on the acceptable use of such practices on the merits of each individual case"[3] (Sherwin, 1989, p. 24). And on the question of abortion in particular, she asserts (controversially) that both standard and feminist medical ethics "accept the need to develop a clear, universal moral policy [favoring unrestricted abortion] so as not to leave space for evaluation on a case by case basis."

But of course, to advocate an absolute or general policy on the basis of any abstract norm or general goal is to deliberately ignore some aspects of context, whether the norm or goal is a feminist one or not. Sherwin argues that the feminist position on abortion is based on "the difference it makes to all women's lives if women are free to decide," and then chides standard medical ethics, in which "policy is formulated in terms of abstract values and rules which are to be invoked whatever the effect on particular persons' lives"[4] (Sherwin, 1989, p. 67). It's hard to understand how a feminist approach like Sherwin's can avoid the same accusation. To advocate an absolute policy because of its liberating effects on all women's lives is to avoid asking what its effects might be on a particular woman's life, unless one is willing to suppose (implausibly) that these liberating effects are universal and invariant, an assumption that would itself repudiate the importance of context.

Take as an another example Sherwin's discussion of the ethics of paternalism. She, like some other feminists, is suspicious of Kantian appeals to rights of individual autonomy, since they are predicated on a masculinist ideal of the isolated, rugged individual. And so, she complains against "philosophic conceptions of autonomy" that they do not fit well with the fact that patients' "decision-making does not always meet the norms that define rationality," leading them to "not. . . always act in accordance with their best interests" (Sherwin, 1992, p. 137).

Yet despite this suspicion, in all that follows she relies utterly on a right of autonomy as the moral bedrock upon which paternalism ultimately founders. The problem with paternalism, she tells us, is that "its actual achievement in bringing about the best consequences is in doubt, because it is the physician's— rather than the patient's—perception of the patient's good that is decisive" (Sherwin, 1992, p. 138). Ultimately, it is the patient who must have the authority to decide, because on the question of what is best, the doctor can claim no objective authority: "The question of the right treatment for a patient is not a question that can be wholly answered by science, because it also involves weighing the patient's own evaluations of the risks and benefits she might experience" (Sherwin, 1992, p. 148).[5] This is a classic argument on behalf of the right of individual choice about matters affecting primarily one's self.

The contrast rings hollow, then, when toward the end of her discussion she asserts that "the ethical question here is not simply a matter of who has a right to make the decision about a patient's health care. . . it is a question of how to strengthen the patient's agency, how to help her make decisions that will serve her well" (Sherwin, 1992, p. 156). The second question presumes that we've answered the first in favor of the patient, and it is the first question and its answer in favor of autonomy that in fact dominates Sherwin's discussion of paternalism.

Another example of this ambivalence toward the use of abstract principles is Susan Wolf's treatment of the issue of assisted suicide. She makes the *de rigueur* denunciation of moral principles:

> "The inadequacies of rights arguments to establish patient entitlement to assisted suicide and euthanasia are linked to the inadequacies of a 'top-down' or deductive bioethics driven by principles, abstract theories or rules. They share certain flaws: both seem overly to ignore context and the nuances of cases; their simple abstractions overlook real power differentials in society and historic subordination; and they avoid the fact that these principles, rules, abstractions and rights are themselves a product of historically oppressive social arrangements."
>
> (Wolf, 1996a, p. 302)

Yet, without reliance on principles, rules, and abstractions (perhaps even historically oppressive ones), Wolf's own arguments against the legalization of assisted suicide would not be possible. To see this, let's start by asking why it is not proper on Wolf's view to speak of a person having a right to assisted death. One of her answers draws an analogy to John Stuart Mill's arguments against the permissibility of voluntarily selling oneself into slavery. "Similarly," Wolf says, "acceding to a patient's request to be killed wipes out the possibility of her future exercise of her liberty" (Wolf, 1996a, p. 301).

But this seems equally true of acceding to a patient's right to refuse life-saving treatment, which Wolf steadfastly defends. Why then does refusal of treatment escape the logic of Wolf's Millean argument against the right to assisted suicide? Because, she tells us, the right to refuse treatment is based in the negative right to be free from bodily invasion, which Wolf insists has no moral connection with any positive right to seek assistance in dying.

What's more, arguments that rely upon invoking our duties to be merciful toward the dying are equally unsuccessful, Wolf contends. First (repeating an argument often made by Leon Kass [1991][6]), assisted death offers only the illusion of mercy, because "no patient is left to experience its supposed benefits."[7] Second, there is no inconsistency in rejecting assisted suicide but permitting the use of pain medications that hasten death, since "the principle of double effect permits giving pain relief and palliative care in doses that risk inducing respiratory depression and thereby hastening death" (Wolf, 1996a, p. 302).

These are all appeals to principles, all of them abstract, absolutist, or both. The right against bodily invasion, for example, is treated as a right that stands on its own, unconnected with more fundamental concerns with empowering self-determination. Hence, the division between negative and positive rights is treated as in principle impermeable, immune from any expectations of consistency. Appealing to a metaphysics of death to refute the claim that assisted suicide may be an act of mercy toward the dying employs a consideration whose relevance can only be of the most abstract kind imaginable, having nothing to do with the experience of those who might think (apparently mistakenly) that they are begging for mercy. And the principle of double effect? Not only a principle of a particularly arcane sort, but one that, in the context employed by Wolf, takes it as absolutely prohibited to deliberately take the life of an innocent person, even with his or her consent. And, I will add, one that has historically been used to narrowly circumscribe the permissibility of abortion.

Feminist writers like Wolf and Sherwin can't have it both ways. They can't both condemn the employment of principles and then use them in their own arguments. But then, as we've seen in earlier chapters, they could hardly avoid using them. Despite their inadequacies, principles seem indispensable for the giving of reasons, and are the medium through which we hold our practices up to our ideals.

The Complexity of Context

Feminists like Sherwin and Wolf also want to extol the overriding importance of context and individual lived experience. Demanding that ethical reflection pay attention to how policy and practice affects all sorts of persons avoids the danger of relying upon pat or conventional assumptions about what "everyone's" experience is like, assumptions that are very likely to be sexist, or blinkered in some other way. On the other hand, in articulating specifically feminist concerns, they must rely in some measure on generalizations about women and their lives in order to support arguments that claim that women as a class of persons are disadvantaged. This introduces a tension that Martha Minow has named the "dilemma of difference" (Minow, 1990, p. 20). For in relying upon generalized claims about what affects women's lives, one risks ignoring the wide variation in the ways these factors manifest themselves in individual cases. And ignoring that variation can unfairly affect those women who don't fit the standard picture.

For example, Wolf starts her essay with concerns about the factors that may systematically disadvantage or endanger women were assisted suicide to be made legal. Among those is recognition of the possibility that women might seek assisted suicide not from a rational assessment of their own interests and considered values, but instead under the spell cast by "the long history of valorizing women's self-sacrifice," a history that has taught women to subjugate their interests to those of others, particularly when those others are men or children (Wolf, 1996a, p. 283). This is a theme she returns to repeatedly as she reviews a series of well-known cases of assisted suicide (Janet Adkins, "Debbie," "Diane," and others), noting that the large majority of Jack Kevorkian's clients were women, and suggesting that this is no mere coincidence:

> "Given this history of images and the valorization of women's self-sacrifice, it should come as no surprise that the early cases dominating the debate about self-sacrifice through physician-assisted suicide and euthanasia have been cases of women."
>
> (Wolf, 1996a, p. 289)

First, let's note that this sentence is a rhetorical sleight of hand. "Self-sacrifice" can be used, as it is in the second half of the sentence, to describe the *act* of suicide (the act being what the debate about the early cases concerned). Or it can be used to characterize the *motive* that someone might have for seeking her own death, which is the sense used in the first half. Wolf here is trying to make it true by definition that women who seek assisted suicide are doing so out of motives of self-sacrifice, which are the products of oppression and thus morally suspicious.

But of course, that is not true by definition. Even given that women as a group are especially vulnerable in the way Wolf describes, it could well be that none of the women she discusses was a slave to traditional feminine virtues of self-sacrifice. Indeed, she produces no specific evidence of such motives for any of them.

If context sensitivity is to be better understood as a method central to feminist ethics, or any ethics for that matter, we need first of all to appreciate that to insist on the importance of "context" is to speak ambiguously, for there are many different sorts and levels of context. When Wolf points out that there is a deeply rooted tradition of self-sacrifice among women, and suggests that this might play a problematic role in some women's decisions to seek assisted suicide, she is expanding our understanding of the *social* context in which a policy concerning assisted suicide will operate. We are now aware of another respect in which some choices for assisted suicide might be less than fully autonomous.

Such awareness hardly amounts to an argument against assisted suicide, because there will be other elements of the social context that also carry moral significance. For example, attention to the social context will also require us to recognize that there are some people, women among them, who are imbued with traditional American values of independence and productivity, and so feel strongly that assisted suicide is the best option for addressing their suffering, which may have little to do with physical pain. And then we will be faced with the question of how to weigh or prioritize these competing considerations. We find ourselves back to the point made above, as well as in our discussion of narrative ethics: increased attention to context will often enrich our appreciation of the complexity of ethical questions, but will not by itself resolve them.

And contexts are not just social; they are also individual, and it is at the level of the individual that multiple social forces are mediated. So it's true that there is a social expectation of feminine self-sacrifice. This is a claim about women as a class. But individual women are not simply "women." They are educated, or not; poor, or not; married, or not; employed, or not; assertive, or not, and so on (with everything in between such simple dichotomies). For this reason, we can't make easy inferences from claims about the social context for policies like those concerning assisted suicide, to conclusions about what meaning or impact these will have at the level of individual choice or action.[8] An analysis informed by understanding of the social or cultural context may not be sufficient if our ethical question concerns a decision being made by an individual.

Take a person like Merian Frederick, one of Kevorkian's patients, whose family founded Merian's Friends after her death to advocate the legalization of assisted suicide in Michigan. Certainly, she was someone who was concerned about the needs of others, and perhaps some of this might be understood to be acting from traditional expectations of women's roles. She expressed the idea that at middle age women "must care for both the young and the old." Despite her age (72), she was the "main support" for her daughter Connie, who had a mild case of phenylketonuria. Watching over Connie "had been [her] occupation, her pride, her motherly instinct." But she was also someone who believed in taking individual responsibility for change, having been an activist in the nuclear disarmament movement. She had always believed in a "planned death for those who are greatly suffering;" and for herself, "wanted control over her life at a time when every day was a struggle to regain control over a lost function." And her concern for others—her impulse to self-sacrifice, if you wish—had an ambivalent quality to it. Perhaps she was concerned about the burden her continued care would place on her family. But her family needed her presence as well, and were themselves torn over her decision to die. Out of consideration for that anguish, "she always tried to weigh her level of comfort against our needs for her." (See Poenisch [1998] for the narrative from which these quotations are drawn.)

No simple explanation can emerge from a complex picture like this. Was Merian Frederick's decision rooted in her notions of motherly self-sacrifice? in her convictions about the suffering person's right to die? in her activist's need to be in control? It could be any, or all of these. Generalizations about gender differences will not much help us understand the dynamics of the decisions that get made by individuals. If we recognize this, we should not be surprised if it turns out that men are more likely to embrace assisted suicide than women are.[9]

The sort of tensions just illustrated between the power of generalizations to help us understand the bigger picture, and the danger they pose of obscuring differences and exceptions that may in fact be more significant in some contexts is at the heart of much contemporary debate within feminism generally.[10] Sometimes attempts to resolve those tensions resemble classical resolutions of the conflict between concern for a general good and respect for individual choice.

An example is provided by Linda LeMoncheck's exposition of a feminist ethics of reproductive health care. After a critical review of Kantian and utilitarian theories, she concludes that neither of these traditional perspectives will motivate providers to empathize with the individual woman's needs or to concern themselves with the political, cultural, and personal forces that may be distorting her capacities for truly informed and free choice.[11] She then recommends a feminist ethics practice that grows out of a "complex and variable dialectic" (LeMoncheck, 1996, p. 170) between a concern that women's use of reproductive technologies not simply perpetuate oppressive control of women's reproductive lives, and the desire to respect the ability of individual women to make choices for themselves that promote and protect their own needs and interests. This dialectic is supported by specific practices, including the requirements that "clinicians spend more time with each patient. . . to discuss the patient's own needs and motivations"; that "clinicians. . . invite each prospective IVF patient to join them in evaluating the most current information concerning the risks, benefits and success rates of IVF for this clinic"; and that provisions be made for "accessible and open forums for the exchange of IVF information and debate, detailing the history of dangerous reproductive experimentation. . . and the ideology of compulsory motherhood, [as well as] information regarding safe and reliable alternatives to IVF" (LeMoncheck, 1996, p. 171). As a result, "clinicians, patients and their families would thus be in a better position to assess the need for, and the benefits of, IVF and embryo transfer, and to allow individual women to make their own decisions as to whether or how such technologies figure in their own lives" (LeMoncheck, 1996, p. 172).

These recommendations can be viewed from two perspectives. From one perspective, they represent a method for resolving the tension between claims about the general dangers and the oppressiveness of reproductive technologies on the one side, and the context-specific needs of individual women on the other. With respect to this purpose, what is specifically feminist about these recommendations is simply the content of some of the recommended materials and activities (e.g., that prospective patients be advised of the history of exploitive experimentation). Otherwise, they seem perfectly on a par with standard liberal reliance on empowering informed individual choice, and with the standard liberal presumption that we should err on the side of permitting too much individual discretion. In these respects, their spirit seems little different than that which insists upon informed consent as a mechanism that permits the benefits of medical research while minimizing the dangers of abuse and exploitation. To the extent that feminist commentators come to similar resolutions to the "dilemma of difference," their *method* is not particularly feminist, however much the object of their moral concern may be.[12]

From another perspective, however, the recommendations aren't really aimed at resolving the tension at all, at least not with respect to justifying any general policy toward reproductive technologies. Instead, they constitute a set of techniques designed to enrich the understandings of the various parties involved. The provider is encouraged to learn more about the needs and motives of her patient; and the patient is encouraged to learn more about the implications of reproductive technology, both personal and political. This may reduce the likelihood that either of them will be acting from superficial motivations, stereotyped assumptions, or the like. This in turn may well reduce the likelihood that individual women will be treated in ways that ignore their needs and capacities for choice. This serves the primary *goal* of a feminist medical ethics, but again, there is nothing particularly feminist about the method itself.

Standpoint Theory

Much the same sort of observations apply to a more systematic attempt to delineate a specifically feminist method sensitive to context—standpoint theory. As Mary Mahowald characterizes it (Mahowald, 1996a), standpoint theory aims to correct our all-too-common ethical myopia.[13] We are nearsighted, because we tend to see the world from our particular perspectives, unaware that others may see and experience it differently. We are too often un-self-conscious about our nearsightedness, and arrogantly assume that our vision is 20/20. And at the social or political level, the nearsightedness of the powerful assumes for itself a universal validity.

The way to correct this myopia is to bring otherwise missing perspectives into the discussion. A feminist standpoint theory will aim to bring out those perspectives of women that have been invisible or brushed aside.

As with the previous discussion of LaMoncheck, we need to ask at this juncture what the goal is of a feminist standpoint theory. Is it a theory that hopes to provide a basis for deciding between competing standpoints? Or is it instead a method for enriching the context of ethical discussion and debate by widening the standpoints that are represented?

For Mahowald it appears to be the latter. Haraway and Hartsock, Mahowald's primary sources, want to privilege the standpoint of the oppressed over that of the dominant group. This is because, in her words, "the standpoints of subjugated groups . . . provide a corrective lens for the myopia of the dominant group." Yet Mahowald then points out that "feminist standpoint theory thus construed cannot adequately reflect all the standpoints of individual women, who, . . . like men, . . . are unique in the compilation of standpoints that each embodies" (Mahowald, 1996a, p. 101). And she later remarks that "nondominant persons are nearsighted also" (Mahowald, 1996a, p. 111). If there is no representing *the* standpoint of the subjugated group, and if even that standpoint can be myopic in its own fashion, then there would seem to be no basis for any systematic or principled privileging of the standpoint of the oppressed.

As with LeMoncheck's feminist reproductive ethics, Mahowald's standpoint theory seems less suited for resolving general questions of policy than for enriching the moral discourse about particular cases. This interpretation of it is supported by Mahowald's examples. In one of them, a woman with phenylketonuria (PKU) is in her second pregnancy and is refusing to follow the phenylalanine-restricted diet that is essential for minimizing the chance that the fetus will inherit an even more severe form of the disease. She also is refusing other interventions intended to reduce this risk to her future child.

Viewed from the perspective of someone without experience of the PKU diet, her attitude may seem irrational or morally perverse, weighing a mere matter of inconvenience or taste over the vital health interests of her fetus. But this perspective may be unable to really appreciate the nature of the burdens on her, as she experiences them. And so, standpoint theory requires that we listen to her account of it and take it seriously. In Mahowald's story, we learn that she had followed these precautions with her first child, but only with great difficulty, leading to the introduction of other sorts of risks to the fetus:

> "Julia [had] attempted to follow the recommended diet, but PKU formulas nauseated her, making it difficult to provide her with sufficient protein to sustain a healthy pregnancy."
>
> (Mahowald, 1996b, p. 338)

And this led in turn to nasogastric feedings at night, and then percutaneous feeding. The result was a child delivered by cesarean section because of intrauterine growth retardation.

It's important to hear this story, because it may help to correct false assumptions about what is being asked of the patient. And indeed, this may in turn serve to turn the weight of ethical argument in favor of not trying to coerce or manipulate the patient into following the diet. But this will not be because the patient's standpoint, being that of a non-dominant person (a patient and a woman), is *per se* privileged. It will be because there remain no other countervailing considerations. But what if we learned that her account of her previous experience was false? Mightn't this undermine the credibility of the standpoint she was representing by it, or at least her claim to in fact occupy such a standpoint? If it did, would we then need to fall back on some more general claim about an individual's right to autonomy, which is not referenced to any particular standpoint? And mightn't we need to have taken some position on the moral relevance of certain other standpoints that might be in conflict with hers? For example, should we consider the standpoint of the child who might be born with maternal PKU? If we do, on what basis do we determine whose standpoint should prevail, or determine what compromises might be ethically made between them?

All of these questions suggest ways in which standpoint theory, however useful a device for enriching our ethical under-standing of a case, will fail to be adequate for justifying any particular resolution of it. Other considerations, of either a principled or non-principled sort, will need to come into play, either to buttress key assumptions or to weigh the moral balance between different standpoints.

A Special Set of Moral Commitments

So far, I've considered two conceptions of a feminist medical ethics. The first takes feminist medical ethics to refer to a goal of inquiry or critique: exposing and reducing the unfair treatment of women. I argued that such a feminist consciousness can be very helpful for surfacing ethically relevant considerations that might otherwise go unnoticed. But since feminist ethics understood in this way focuses on only one particular category of moral concerns, it cannot by itself constitute an adequate medical ethic.

The second conception sees feminist medical ethics as a method of inquiry, in particular one that abjures the use of abstract moral principle, and extols the significance of particular contexts. This is a false contrast in several ways. First, even those feminists who employ this rhetoric cannot seem to avoid the use of abstract principle. In part, this is because some level of generalization is necessary for interpreting the moral significance of various features of the context. Second, there are always multiple contexts to be accommodated, whether between different individuals or classes of individuals, or within the life of a single person. "Context" as a tool of moral discourse can do little to negotiate among the competing moral considerations these various contexts introduce. Still, the notion of context is useful for underscoring our individual moral myopia, and the corresponding need to expand the range of participants and perspectives engaged in moral conversation.

In this section, I will examine a third conception: feminist ethics as a special set of moral commitments or norms.

This third form of feminist ethics is most commonly referred to as an "ethics of care." The feminist use of it, at least, originates in Carol Gilligan's study of moral development, *In A Different Voice*. In that book, Gilligan claims to have found that women tend to speak and think of their moral commitments differently than men:

> "The moral imperative that emerges repeatedly in interviews with women is an injunction to care, a responsibility to discern and alleviate the 'real and recognizable trouble' of this world. For men, the moral imperative appears

rather as an injunction to respect the rights of others and thus to protect from interference the rights to life and self-fulfillment."

(Gilligan, 1993, 100)

This difference is reflected, Gilligan claims, in women's greater concern with establishing and maintaining particular relationships with those around them, as contrasted with men's greater emphasis on abstract rights and duties that lie beyond individual ties or affections.

Caring: Neither Feminine Nor Feminist?

Gilligan's claims about a special female moral voice are often taken at face value, when they are as an empirical matter highly controversial. Christine Gudorf, for example, claims that "[Gilligan's] research has demonstrated that instead of relying (as Kohlberg had shown morally mature males do) on abstract moral principles as the guides for discrete, autonomous individuals, females attempt to make pragmatic choices that safeguard the persons and relationships about which they care" (Gudorf, 1994, pp. 165–166; my emphasis).[14]

Gilligan herself has usually been more modest.[15] The evidence in fact is not so categorical as Gudorf and others portray it. There is, to begin with, considerable room for interpreting the responses of Gilligan's informants in ways significantly different than hers, so that responses that she encodes as examples of a "care" ethic might be counted as examples of appeals to principles or rights, and vice versa. (See Jonathan Dancy [1991] for discussion of this.) The other problem is that subsequent research in comparative moral development, some of it by Gilligan's colleagues, has failed to confirm any clear or consistent gender differences in moral orientation. In his excellent critical review of the literature, Owen Flanagan concludes that "much of the data now emerging points to the psychological reality of the different voice in many boys and men as well as in girls and women. . . nothing like the stark early difference claims can be defended" (Flanagan, 1991, p. 228).

A health care-related example of such research is reported by Kuhse and Singer (1997), in which they presented a set of moral dilemmas to groups of physicians and nurses. For each situation, sets of alternative reasons or considerations were developed, and coded for whether they were "partialist" ("care") or "impartialist" ("justice") in their orientation. Subjects were asked to identify the sorts of reasons or considerations most significant to them in deciding what they would do. On analysis, there was no association between the subjects' employment of partialist- or care-oriented reasons and their profession, their sex, or their score on a scale of masculinity/femininity.

Thus, although there may well be "different voices" in which people speak of their ethical concerns, there is no reason to think that any one of those voices belongs especially to women.

Another difficulty, pointed out by some feminists, is that even if the ethic of care were a distinctively feminine ethic, it would not be a good model for a *feminist* ethic that was concerned with the oppression of women. As it is usually represented, a care ethic features an overriding commitment to sustaining relationships, and being sensitive and responsive to the needs of others. These are disturbingly like the traditional feminine virtues that serve to keep women in the service of men and children. (See Kuhse, 1997, Chapter 2, for a good overview of the history of the traditional feminine virtues, and their appropriation by nursing.) As Susan Sherwin puts it, "the nurturing and caring at which women excel are, among other things, the survival skills of an oppressed group that lives in close contact with its oppressors" (Sherwin, 1992, 50).

What is an Ethics of Care?

Even if, for the reasons given above, an ethic of care is not a specifically feminist ethic, it might still be a distinctive and viable model for ethical deliberation. This gets us to the heart of the difficulty with an ethics of care: either it is not distinctive, or it is not viable.

On the matter of the care ethic's distinctiveness, it is first of all important to argue that the contrasts commonly drawn between an ethic of care and an ethic of justice or principles are false ones. Extensive critical discussion of commonly made contrasts can be found in Kuhse (1997, esp. Chapter 6) and in Dancy (1992). A few examples will be enough to illustrate the nature of the difficulty.

One contrast has it that the ethics of care is concerned to be sensitive to the particular context, as opposed to an ethics of justice or duty, which is applied abstractly without regard to specific circumstances. As Dancy points out, however, Ross' theory of *prima facie* duties requires attention to all of the moral concerns arising out of a particular situation, and urges the decision that best preserves as many of them as possible under the specific circumstances.[16] Like the care theorist, Ross rejects the idea that an ethical solution can be derived from any set of principles in the abstract. This is true as well of utilitarianism, which requires sensitivity to context in order to best inform a judgment about the course of action that will yield the best consequences—under the circumstances.[17]

To take another, it is often claimed that an ethic of care is partialist, and thus concerned foremost with the needs of those nearest and dearest; while an ethic of justice or principle is impartialist, and so must be unaffected by the ethical pull of human emotion and relationships. But again, a Rossian set of *prima facie* duties will include many that are specific to particular kinds of relationships (there are traditionally duties of friendship, marriage, parenthood, and so on). And since deep human feelings will inform of any vision of human good, utilitarians will also want to accommodate them: there are good utilitarian reasons for recognizing special obligations of parents to their children.

The source of misleading contrasts like these is the tendency of care theorists to use a particularly rigid species of Kantianism as their stalking horse, forgetting that there are a number of other ways in which to understand the role of moral principles and the demands of impartiality and universalizability. Even Kant is not fairly treated, since it is often forgotten that he offered a second version of the categorical imperative: "Act so that you treat humanity, whether in your own person or in that of another, always as an end and never as a means only" (Kant, 1959, p. 47). It would not be implausible to interpret this as requiring that one be concerned for and respectful of the ends of others, and this requires a sensitive appreciation of others as individuals. Dancy observes that even if Kantian legislators are thin rational agents, those who must be treated fairly are not, and it would then "be impossible to operate the justice perspective successfully without a sympathetic knowledge of their feelings, hopes and fears" (Dancy, 1992, p. 451). Human sympathy might well be a Kantian virtue, but such a complicating possibility is left out of many care theorists' accounts.

Here a care theorist might acknowledge that one or another more traditional ethical theory can accommodate one or another of the defining themes of the care ethic. But what they don't do is take the injunction to care as their first principle, where this is to be understood as Noddings (1984) understands it—not as the application of an axiom in a rational system, but rather as an ethical ideal expressed through an "affective-receptive" mode of interaction with someone in need.

The trouble is that "caring," whether understood as a principle, an ethical ideal, or a virtue of character, is by itself too inchoate a notion to provide much ethical direction. As an ethical ideal it is always parasitic on other ethical commitments. This is because, as Peter Allmark points out, the invitation to care leaves entirely open what we should care about; who we should care about, or how we should express our care. People can and commonly do care about all sorts of reprehensible things and despicable people, and are led by that caring to do things that are ethically objectionable. To allude to an example that Noddings uses,[18] one might care for only one's white brothers, not the blacks who live on the next block, and be led to fight on behalf of a racist regime. What's more, the virtues often associated with an ethic of care—of sensitivity, responsiveness, discernment, and so on—are ethical virtues only when yoked to some credible vision of the good and of right action. Someone who makes his living as a con man can be careful and skillful in his work, employing skills of sensitivity, responsiveness, and discernment. Presumably the virtues of a good con man are not thereby ethical virtues.

This means that an ethic of care can never act alone. An example illustrating this is a discussion by the nurse Randy Spreen Parker, who intends to illustrate the ethic of care with the story of one of her patients. Mike's severe diabetes, emphysema, and a stroke have left him a double amputee and aphasic, with difficulty speaking coherently or understanding others. Despite these problems and being confined to a nursing home, Mike seemed to be doing well until recurring infection required removal of his right femur and the surrounding tissue. Parker became his nurse after surgery. Affected by what clearly seems to be his severe pain and distress caused by unending dressing changes and debridements of infected tissue, she undertakes to learn how to communicate with Mike nonverbally. Through this "dialogue,"

Parker claims, "it became clear to us both that dressing changes and further medical interventions served no meaningful purpose" (Parker, 1990, p. 33).

This leads her to approach the attending physician to inform him that Mike no longer wants life-sustaining treatment. But, Parker recounts, "I tried to explain my rationale but found myself struggling for the right words. How could I translate my own moral experience into traditional moral language?" (Parker, 1990, p. 33). She concludes that since she can't, her "experience with Mike suggests that the values essential to the moral foundation of nursing cannot be extracted from any abstract or decontextualized moral theory" (Parker, 1990, p. 34).

But of course she has already translated her moral experience, into the language of patient self-determination. It is because she attaches value to (cares about) the views of the patient that she is concerned to discover what he feels and wants. It is because she cares about his right to control what is happening to him more than she cares about sustaining his life (the sanctity of life view she attributes to the others caring for him) that she is moved to do something on his behalf. And it is because she thinks that his wishes are an overriding value that she thinks it ethically germane to report to the attending physician what she thinks those wishes are.

Far from shunning reliance on any "abstract" moral theory, Parker depends upon one. She couldn't do otherwise. For her caring response to have any ethical direction or significance, it must be responsive not to everything and anything, but to those things that matter ethically. Which things those are presupposes some hierarchy of purposes, consequences, and obligations. That hierarchy originates outside the caring response itself.

The ethics of care, then, is not a viable method or perspective for ascertaining right choices. What remains are the *virtues* of caring, which become ethical virtues when tied to some credible normative ethic. Care theorists are right to emphasize such virtues as responsiveness, sensitivity, and discernment, because these capacities are necessary for implementing any ethic. These and other virtues, and their connection to the non-inferential judgments that are pervasive in moral deliberation, will be the subject of the next chapter.

Notes

1. Much the same claim about core feminism is made by others as well, including Susan Sherwin—"[All feminist ethics] share some political analysis of the unequal power between men and women" (Sherwin, 1989, p. 22); Susan Wolf—"feminist work ... seeks to understand . . . and strives to change the distribution and use of power to stop the oppression of women" (Wolf, 1996b, p. 8); and Mary Mahowald—"the ethical criterion for determining the relevance of differences between women and men is gender justice or equality" (Mahowald, 1996a, p. 95).

2. Although in fact I am not convinced, because I don't think the authors mount a compelling argument against the possibility that parental duties to care might responsibly be transferred.

3. Note that Linda LaMoncheck, discussed below, insists that a feminist reproductive ethics should insist on judging women's employment of reproductive technologies on precisely a case-by-case basis.

4. This hyperbole is obviously false.

5. These sorts of arguments, of course, didn't originate in feminism, and have been stock in trade of conventional medical ethics at least since Robert Veatch.

6. For example, "Can one benefit the patient as a whole by making him dead? There is, of course, a logical difficulty: how can any good exist for a being that is not?" (Kass, 1991, p. 10).

7. This is an ironic twist on the old Stoic argument that death was not an evil to be feared because upon death there was no longer any person to suffer the evil.

8. See Blacksher's (1998) and Labacqz' (1998) discussions for more on the dangers of generalizing or essentializing difference.

9. See Ganzini et al. (1998), whose study indicated that men with ALS were more likely to want to have the assisted suicide option.

10. See Bordo (1989) for a discussion that tries to rescue the significance and usefulness of generalizations about women's experience from the postmodernist insistence on ferreting out difference.

11. I find these arguments unpersuasive, on the whole, because they rest on crude and stereotyped characterizations of these traditions. She claims, for example, that "there is no requirement in an ethics of utility that the clinician ask the patient for her understanding of the short- or long-term benefits of undergoing IVF" (LeMoncheck, 1996, p. 169). This is a claim that is hard to credit if the ethics of utility takes individual preferences to be the good that should be maximized. A preference utilitarian would be duty-bound to inquire into the patient's own understandings and values.

12. For another example, see Kirkland and Tong (1996), who rely upon a "deliberative model" of informed consent to allow for the possibility of feminist cosmetic surgery.

13. Mahowald borrows much of her account of standpoint theory from Donna Haraway (1988) and Nancy C. M. Hartsock (1985).

14. See also Virginia Held (1990, p. 331) and Susan Sherwin (1989, p. 18; 1992, p. 46).

15. In the Preface to *A Different Voice*, she cautions that "The different voice I describe is characterized not by gender but by theme. Its association with women is an empirical observation ... But this association is not absolute" (Gilligan, 1993, p. 2).

16. Explicating Ross, Dancy says that "our decision in a particular case is not reached by subsuming what we find here under a moral principle, but by looking as carefully as we can at the ways in which the features that matter here go together ... there is no suggestion that the only approach possible is one likely to generate firm answers" (Dancy, 1992, p. 457).

17. Kuhse (1997) discusses the importance of context, and the utilitarian use of it, at p. 122 ff.

18. See her discussion of Ms. A in Noddings, 1984, pp. 109–113.

Bibliography

Andrews, Lori. 1988. "Surrogate Motherhood: The Challenge for Feminists." *Law, Medicine and Health Care* 16(1-2):72–80.

Allmark, Peter. 1995. "Can There Be an Ethics of Care?" *Journal of Medical Ethics* 21:19–24.

Blacksher, Erika. 1998. "Desperately Seeking Difference." *Cambridge Quarterly of Healthcare Ethics* 7:11–16.

Bordo, Susan. 1989. "Feminism, Postmodernism, and Gender-Skepticism." In *Feminism/Postmodernism*, ed. Linda J. Nicholson. New York: Routledge.

Dancy, Jonathan. 1992. "Caring About Justice." *Philosophy* 67:447–466.

Flanagan, Owen. 1991. *Varieties of Moral Personality: Ethics and Psychological Realism*. Cambridge: Harvard University Press.

Ganzini, Linda, Wendy S. Johnson, Bentson H. McFarland, et al. 1998. "Attitudes of Patients with Amyotrophic Lateral Sclerosis and Their Care Givers toward Assisted Suicide." *New England Journal of Medicine* 339:967–973.

Gilligan, Carol. 1993. *In a Different Voice: Psychological Theory and Women's Development*. Cambridge: Harvard University Press.

Gudorf, Christine E. 1994. "A Feminist Critique of Biomedical Principlism." In *A Matter of Principles? Ferment in U.S. Bioethics*. Ed. Edwin R. Dubose, Ronald P. Hamel and Laurence J. O'Connell. Valley Forge, PA: Trinity Press International, pp. 164–181.

Haraway, Donna. 1988. "Situated Knowledges: The Science Question in Feminism and the Privilege of Partial Perspective." *Feminist Studies* 14:575–599.

Hartsock, Nancy C. M. 1985. *Money, Sex and Power: Toward a Feminist Historical Materialism*. Boston: Northeastern University Press.

Held, Virginia. 1990. "Feminist Transformations of Moral Theory." *Philosophy and Phenomenological Research*. Vol. 1 (Supplement): 321–344

Jaggar, Alison M. 1991. "Feminist Ethics: Projects, Problems, Prospects." In *Feminist Ethics*, ed. Claudia Card. Lawrence, KS: University Press of Kansas, pp. 78–104.

Kant, Immanuel. 1959. *Foundations of the Metaphysics of Morals*. Trans. Lewis White Beck. Indianapolis: Bobbs-Merrill.

Kass, Leon R. 1991. "Why Doctors Must Not Kill." *Commonweal* 118, no. 14 (Supplement):8–12.

Kirkland, Anna and Rosemarie Tong. 1996. "Working within Contradiction: The Possibility of Feminist Cosmetic Surgery." *Journal of Clinical Ethics* 7(2, Summer):151–159.

Kuhse, Helga. 1997. *Caring: Nurses, Women and Ethics*. Oxford: Blackwell Publishers.

Kuhse, Helga and Peter Singer, 1997. "Partial and impartial ethical reasoning in health care professionals." *Journal of Medical Ethics* 23:226–232.

Lebacqz, Karen. 1998. "Difficult Difference." *Cambridge Quarterly of Healthcare Ethics* 7:17–26.

LeMoncheck, Linda. 1996. "Philosophy, Gender Politics, and In Vitro Fertilization: A Feminist Ethics of Reproductive Health Care." *Journal of Clinical Ethics* 7(2, Summer):160–176.

Mahowald, Mary. 1996a. "On Treatment of Myopia: Feminist Standpoint Theory and Bioethics." In *Feminism and Bioethics: Beyond Reproduction*, Ed. Susan M. Wolf. New York: Oxford University Press, pp. 95–116.

Mahowald, Mary. 1996b. "A Feminist Standpoint for Genetics." *Journal of Clinical Ethics* 7(4, Winter):333–340.

Minow, Martha. 1990. *Making All The Difference: Inclusion, Exclusion and American Law*. Ithaca: Cornell University Press.

Nelson, Hilde Lindemann and Nelson James Lindeman 1989. "Cutting Motherhood in Two: Some Suspicions Concerning Surrogacy." *Hypatia* 4(3):85–95. Reprinted in *Feminist Perspectives in Medical Ethics*, ed. Helen Bequaert Holmes and Laura M. Purdy. Bloomington: Indiana University Press, 1992.

Nelson, Hilde Lindemann and Nelson James Lindeman. 1996. "Justice in the Allocation of Health Care Resources: A Feminist Account." In *Feminism and Bioethics: Beyond Reproduction*, Ed. Susan M.Wolf. New York: Oxford University Press, pp. 351–370.

Noddings, Nel. 1984. *Caring: A Feminine Approach to Ethics and Moral Education*. Berkeley: University of California Press.

Parker, Randy Spreen. 1990. "Nurses' Stories: The Search for a Relational Ethic of Care." *Advances in Nursing Science* 13:31–40.

Pierce, Christine. 1991. "Postmodernism and Other Skepticisms." In *Feminist Ethics*, ed. Claudia Card. Lawrence, Kansas: University of Kansas Press.

Poenisch, Carol. 1998. "Merian Frederick's Story." *New England Journal of Medicine* 339:996–998.

Purdy, Laura M. 1996. *Reproducing Persons: Issues in Feminist Bioethics*. Ithaca: Cornell University Press.

Sherwin, Susan. 1989. "Feminist and Medical Ethics: Two Different Approaches to Contextual Ethics." *Hypatia* 4(2):57–72.

Sherwin, Susan. 1992. *No Longer Patient: Feminist Ethics and Health Care*. Philadelphia: Temple University Press.

Wolf, Susan. 1996a. "Gender, Feminism and Death: Physician-Assisted Suicide and Euthanasia." In Susan Wolf. *Feminism and Bioethics: Beyond Reproduction*. New York: Oxford University Press, pp. 282–317.

Wolf, Susan. 1996b. "Introduction: Gender and Feminism in Bioethics." In Susan Wolf. *Feminism and Bioethics: Beyond Reproduction*. New York: Oxford University Press, pp. 3–46.

Chapter 7

Virtue Theory

So far in our discussion, we've focused on methods for deciding what we should do in choosing among alternative actions or policies. Our ordinary moral discourse, however, is concerned not just with what we should do, but also with what sort of persons we should be. We expect ourselves and others to possess a minimal set of common virtues like honesty and kindness. We admire those who have developed traits like courage to an especially high degree. And we may have special, or especially stringent, expectations for those working in health care—that they be compassionate, say, or altruistic.

That we have a vocabulary of the virtues, and that health professionals are expected to possess special virtues may be obvious enough. It's a more controversial matter what the relation is between the possession of virtue and the making of right choices. Are these two separate realms of moral discourse? If these are not two wholly separate realms, how are they connected? What, for example, is the connection between virtues and principles or rules? Can a virtue ethics substitute for an ethics of principles and rules? Less radically, are virtues a necessary adjunct to a rule-based ethics? Or are virtues at best a means for encouraging right conduct? And how might the answers to these questions affect our approaches to ethical issues in health care?

The Attractions of Virtue

Modern proponents advocate attention to virtue for several different sorts of reasons, which are important to distinguish.

Some see the virtues, or at least some of them, as necessary conditions for our knowledge of the right choice. The most common variant of this view takes virtues to be epistemic *powers* by which we are able to grasp the right choice, suited to each particular set of circumstances. On this conception, virtues are a vehicle for ethical knowledge that transcends the limitations of rules or principles. For most modern exponents of this idea, Aristotle provides the model. Aristotle understood right choices to issue from a good character, capable of choosing the best means to achieving human excellence and happiness. The courageous person, for instance, makes choices that are neither rash at one extreme, nor cowardly at the other, but at the proper place in between. That proper balance is not specifiable by any rule but is a product of a practical wisdom (*phronesis*) that unites intellectual and moral virtues. The judgment depends, as Aristotle says, "on particular facts, and the decision rests with perception," rather than rule (Aristotle, 1941, 1109b23).

Some such capacity seems necessary if, as we've seen throughout this book, principles by themselves always underdetermine our moral choices. If principles alone are inadequate for moral knowledge, some degree of ethical skepticism seems unavoidable unless our moral judgments can be warranted by something other than, or more than, discursive reasons. For many, virtue appears to offer this firewall against skepticism.

It is appreciation of the limits of universally valid principles that leads philosophers like John McDowell to insist that "Occasion by occasion, one knows what to do (if one does) not by applying universal principles but by being a certain kind of person: one who sees situations in a certain distinctive way" (McDowell, 1989, p. 105).

McDowell seems to think of reliance on virtue as a replacement for reliance on rule. A less radical alternative is to see it as a necessary supplement to principle—virtue is the tool by which principles and rules are applied. This is the view embraced by Pellegrino and Thomasma, who insist that "good dispositions or good character alone will not ensure that the act or moral choice is good. . . Moral principles are the benchmarks against which we may assess the moral quality of [acts]" (Pellegrino and Thomasma, 1993, p. 21). For them, virtues play a "mediating" role between conflicting principles, enabling the agent to apply such principles for the best under the circumstances (Pellegrino and Thomasma, 1993, p. 27).

These epistemic roles are not the only ones into which virtues have been cast. Instead of seeing them as powers, one might see them as *dispositions* that motivate, rather than determine, the right choices. This is probably the sense of "virtue" with which we are most familiar. The "fair" person does not merely know in some detached way what fairness requires; she is consistently inclined to act in accordance with the demands of fairness. She adopts fairness as a personal commitment, and this commitment is a moral excellence in her. To say she is fair is not just to commend her actions; it is to commend her as a person.

Pellegrino and Thomasma see virtue playing this dispositional role as well. It is the role foremost in mind when they advocate a return to virtue in medicine. "The most crucial dilemmas of medical ethics today are. . . dilemmas of professional ethics, [which] must reconcile two opposing orders—one based on the primacy of its covenant with patients and the other based on the ethos of self-interest" (Pellegrino and Thomasma, 1993, p. 31). Thus, "the imperative most central to being a profession and indispensable for medical morality [is] effacement of self-interest" (Pellegrino and Thomasma, 1993, p. 42). The virtues are valuable not only epistemically, but instrumentally, because they increase the likelihood of physicians acting rightly (i.e., in accordance with their obligations to patients).

This distinction between epistemic and dispositional roles for virtue has several important features. When virtues are epistemic moral powers, possession of virtues (some or all of them) is at least a necessary (and perhaps also a sufficient) condition for knowing the right thing to do. The contrast between a "virtue ethics" and a "rule ethics" is that the latter is a defective theory of moral knowledge. But when virtues are thought of as dispositions rather than powers, no such contrast follows. Even an ethics that warrants moral knowledge entirely by appeal to rules will still be interested, as a practical matter, in understanding and cultivating the traits of mind and character that most encourage proper conformance with the moral rules. Martha Nussbaum (1999) points out that most of the great modern moralists, including Bentham, Kant, Mill, and others, published substantial discussions of the virtues even though their moral theories were not virtue-based. When we conceive of virtues as dispositions, they need not also be necessary conditions for *knowing* what to do (although they may remain motivationally necessary for *actually doing* the right thing).

In assessing arguments for any "virtue theory," we need to be careful not to conflate these two roles. In particular, reasons that convince us of the importance of cultivating virtues as dispositions may give us no reason whatsoever to think that virtues play any essential epistemic role in moral deliberation. The possibility of such a confusion lurks in Pellegrino and Thomasma's claim that "the virtues are conditions of possibility for the implementation of principles and moral rules" (Pellegrino and Thomasma, 1993, p. 28). Are they speaking of the material or the logical possibility? I will discuss below whether their discussion mistakes one for the other.

There are two possible roles for virtues in our moral thinking, then: virtues as powers necessary for knowing the right choices, and virtues as dispositions that reflect the moral excellence of persons. I will argue below that the first role for virtue cannot be defended, but the second offers a supplementary perspective not just on character, but on choices as well, that is practically useful in health care ethics.

Virtues as Powers

If virtues are powers of moral knowledge, the question arises what sort of power this is. What is the relationship between having virtue, and having knowledge of the right thing to do? Here there are two possibilities. One is simply to define "right choice" in terms of what the virtuous person would do. According to Rosalind Hursthouse, in virtue theories, "An action is right iff [if and only if] it is what a virtuous agent would do in the circumstances" (Hursthouse, 1997, p. 219). The relationship is a *logical* one, which we might dub the "logical power of virtue."

The alternative is to think of virtue in the terms discussed earlier—as offering a special kind of perception, the ability to "see" what is right. The relationship is an *epistemic* one, which we might dub the "perceptual power of virtue."

I'll discuss this second alternative a bit later. Let's start with the first one: Is it plausible to think that "Choice X is the right choice" *means* "Choice X is what the virtuous person would do"? There are a number of reasons to think not.

The Logical Power of Virtue

First, how would we decide, from the alternatives in front of us, which was the right or best choice? We'd first have to know which persons were virtuous, or virtuous enough, and then inquire which choice they would make.[1] But how would we identify the virtuous? Is it by their acts that we would know them? Then we would identify virtuous persons by identifying those among us who choose rightly, at least most of the time.

But this account of the matter would make virtue irrelevant to our knowledge of right choices, since it assumes we can know which choices are the right ones before we know who the virtuous are. Right choices could not be defined as those the virtuous person would make without falling into a trivial circularity. Indeed this account would see the logical connection running entirely in the other direction: to say that someone is virtuous is merely to say that he habitually chooses rightly.

If the logical priority of virtue is to remain a substantive position, it will have to propose some other route by which the virtuous are known. Hursthouse argues for one such alternative. Starting with the premise cited earlier, she adds that "A virtuous agent is one who acts virtuously, that is, one who has and exercises the virtues," and then that "A virtue is a character trait a human being needs to flourish or live well." (Hursthouse, 1997, p. 219). This avoids trivial circularity, but it does so by making virtue theory a kind of foundationalism—acts are judged by their relationship to an ultimate value: human well-being or happiness (*eudaimonia*). Virtue does not occupy a position of logical priority, and claims no special epistemic role in warranting moral knowledge. Hursthouse's virtue theory might well be defensible, but in it virtues are conceived as excellences, rather than powers, and so it will be discussed further below.

One other method for identifying the virtuous remains. Traditionally, virtue was identified with the occupants of certain social classes or roles: the aristocrat, the gentleman, the cleric, the doctor. Perhaps if we could count on the virtue of such persons, without needing to examine their specific choices, then our virtue theory could at least avoid circularity. But this is a quaint suggestion in a world as insistently egalitarian as ours (in its rhetoric, if not its reality). We are hard put to place our faith in any class of persons, whose goodness and rectitude we trust implicitly. Physicians are a particularly prominent example of this. The whole point of the patients' rights movement that began in the 1960s, and that continues unabated to this day, is to challenge the moral authority of physicians. That challenge is based on the perception that physicians (along with most other figures of social authority) are not paragons of virtue, but as flawed as the rest of us, a perception fueled by recurring scandals revealing the willingness of some physicians to sacrifice the interests of patients (see the discussions by Rothman [1991] and Katz [1984], among many others).

In the absence of any other defensible account of who the virtuous are, the thesis that right conduct might be defined as what the virtuous would choose either degenerates into circularity, or relies on an antiquated elitism at odds with the facts of professional conduct.

The Perceptual Power of Virtue

Perhaps the alternative is more promising—virtue consists in, or confers, an epistemic power of moral perception. This is the sense attached to Aristotle's master virtue, *phronesis*, commonly translated as "prudence." It is the skill, or practical wisdom, of knowing what is best to do in a particular set of circumstances, where rules or principles can offer only rough, or conflicting, guidance. For Pellegrino and Thomasma, prudence is the medium connecting rules with particular choices. "Prudence enables us to discern which means are most appropriate to the good in particular circumstances" (Pellegrino and Thomasma, 1993, p. 84). Although rules are essential elements in our moral thinking, they cannot be expected to account for the infinite variety of real-life circumstances. In "complex clinical decisions," Pellegrino and Thomasma say,

> "the answers given in the abstract or as an exercise in balancing prima facie principles against one other [sic] might seem simpler than they are in practice. Here again we confront the need for moral insight, for that combination of intuitive grasp by natural inclination of what is right and good here, and how in this decision we call prudence to resolve these conflicts in ways no formula can guarantee."
>
> (Pellegrino and Thomasma, 1993, p. 89)

They give a number of examples where prudence is necessary for making these particular judgments. Regarding the process of getting patient consent, they ask:

> "When does obtaining consent become coercive? When should the physician try to persuade, and when is he unduly influencing the decision? Is it not tantamount to moral abandonment not to advise the patient on the basis of our best estimate of the interests of the patient? Yet if we express our own preferences, do we not subtly overmaster the vulnerable patient? The prudent physician is the one we expect to make these difficult distinctions on the basis of a character fixed in its disposition to act well, to keep the end of healing in its totality in view, and to

modulate the application of means so as to foster but not frustrate that end."

(Pellegrino and Thomasma, 1993, p. 88)

This account prompts several points. First, we need to remember the distinction between virtues as powers and virtues as dispositions to act rightly. In this passage, as in other places throughout, Pellegrino and Thomasma link their epistemic characterization of the "prudent" physician with the dominant theme of their book—a call for the reinvigoration of medical virtues, especially the virtue of self-effacement, as a trustworthy set of dispositions to act in accordance with a principle of patient interest, rather than self-interest. As I've pointed out, however, it's wrong to think that our hearty agreement with them on this latter point implies something about the nature or necessity of "prudence," or any other virtue, as a prerequisite for moral knowledge. Pellegrino and Thomasma repeatedly invite this fallacy, even if they don't explicitly commit it.

Second, although they've insisted on the indispensability of principles, here as in their other examples, they have little to say about just where or how principles and prudence link up. Surely it can't be the case that prudence is all that's required to answer the sort of questions posed in the example cited. A principled analysis would have a lot to say about what counts as "undue influence" or "moral abandonment."[2] Presumably, since their brand of *phronesis* is not billed as a top-to-bottom intuitionism, prudence would come into play where principles were exhausted. This would be exactly the territory mapped, with particular examples, in earlier chapters of the present book, where moral reflection requires judgment in the balancing or interpretation of principle. And this would appear to be the scope of "prudence" suggested by Pellegrino and Thomasma's characterization of it.

And this gets us to the third point. Why should we think that prudence is capable of playing this epistemic role? The argument on behalf of virtue's epistemic necessity is a negative one. In this, Pellegrino and Thomasma echo other writers, like John McDowell (cited earlier) and Alasdair MacIntyre (1984): The decisions we need to make in particular cases cannot be warranted entirely by appeals to rules; yet we can and must make them; therefore, these decisions are warranted by something in addition to rules; and this something is properly called virtue or prudence.

The argument is unsatisfactory on two counts. First, it assumes that the decisions forced on us by circumstances must be entirely warranted by *some* form of knowledge. If knowledge of principles alone is not enough, there must be some other kind of knowledge taking up the slack. An alternative assumption, however, is that such decisions simply step beyond the bounds of justification, even if in some respects they may be constrained by them—that is, there is nothing available to take up the slack. To rule out this alternative, the virtue theorist must be able to respond with an argument that shows how virtue or prudence carries the needed epistemic power. But that argument cannot be the negative one we're discussing, since it's the soundness of that very argument that's up for grabs. What's needed instead is a positive argument that explains, rather than assumes, the epistemic power of prudence.

That power can't be claimed by a question-begging stipulation, as Pellegrino and Thomasma do: "Prudence is an essential element of the clinical judgment because prudence is, to repeat St. Aquinas' trenchant phrase, a *recto ratio agibilium*—a right way of acting." (Pellegrino and Thomasma, 1993, p. 90). But when writers try to do more than this, they are drawn into a principle-driven discourse. Ulrik Kihlbom, for example, claims that "What make some actions morally right are the factors the virtuous person perceives in the situation as morally relevant" (Kihlbom, 2000, p. 290), and so he agrees that the proper exercise of virtue requires "apprehending the reason that something is morally right or wrong" (Kihlbom, 2000, p. 301).

What form would such reasons take? Are they matters of my private moral "perception," the sort of thing only other virtuous folks can apprehend? This doesn't explain virtue's epistemic power; it leaves it a mystery. It also offers no language for adjudicating disagreements between equally virtuous persons.[3]

More plausibly, those reasons must refer to features of the situation observable by others, at least potentially, and this is the option that Kihlbom prefers. And so he argues that the virtuous nurse who "sees" that it is wrong to continue aggressively treating a patient "did not just experience the wrongness: full stop."[4] For her perception to count as moral knowledge, she must be able to say things like:

> "The patient is in severe pain and suffers immensely, he won't live for much longer even with the life-sustaining treatment, something he is well aware of. Knowing him well, I'm convinced that he wants to end the treatment. This is why the treatment ought to be ended." (Kihlbom, 2000, p. 302)

These read like just the sorts of things that might be said by someone appealing to principles, whether in a foundationalist, pluralist, or coherentist framework.[5] If this is how its epistemic power is explained, then virtue contributes nothing to our capacities for moral knowledge.

The second problem with the negative argument on behalf of virtue's power arises even if we're willing to grant that there must be something doing the epistemic work not done by principles, and willing to call it "prudence." What has this added to our understanding of moral reflection, or to our capacity to more fully justify our moral choices? The answer, I'm afraid, is still nothing. "Prudence" becomes an impenetrable black box, and its invocation only so much hand-waving. Rather than pointing to a deepened understanding of moral deliberation, it's a label for what we can't further explain. This inarticulateness about "prudence" began with Aristotle: "virtue, then, is a state of character concerned with choice, lying on a mean, i.e., the mean relative to us, this being determined by a rational principle, and by that principle by which the man of practical wisdom would determine it" (Aristotle, 1941, 1107a). What the "principle" is Aristotle does not say—it's whatever principle operates when prudence is properly exercised. The inarticulateness continues with modern exponents of virtue theory: "The prudent physician or patient is the one who can order habitually fact and principle more sensitively and correctly to each other and act appropriately to achieve the good of the patient" (Pellegrino and Thomasma, 1993, p. 23). How prudence gauges choices "more sensitively and correctly," or how we know that it has achieved such results, is not further explained.

Here, no doubt, advocates of virtue theory will remind us of Aristotle's dictum that we should expect no more exactitude than the subject matter will allow. Precisely. Instead of empty talk about "prudence," it would be better to remain silent. This is not to dismiss the significance of the problem presented by the necessity of judgment in moral decision-making. What can we conclude, then, about the "power" of virtue? The logical power of virtue can find no good escape from trivial circularity. And the perceptual power of virtue remains something more asserted than explained. Perhaps virtue's other role will fare better.

Virtues as Moral Excellences

In its second role, virtue claims no special power, but claims instead a special moral territory—those characteristics that make persons morally better or worse. Which characteristics these are has depended on the era and the culture. The Greeks listed fortitude, temperance, justice, and wisdom as the cardinal moral virtues; the Christians added faith, hope, and charity. Virtues like these might be taken to apply to all persons; other virtues might be linked to, or emphasized by, a particular role or class of persons. Pellegrino and Thomasma argue that virtues like fidelity and self-effacement are especially important for physicians. This cultural and role relativity leads Robert Veatch to remark that "It is not going too far to say that one could have virtually any set of virtues one wanted for the physician by simply picking the cultural tradition and time period properly" (Veatch, 1985, p. 334).

Which Virtues?

Thus, the first question facing us is how we can know which virtues and vices to include in our appraisals. The difficulty in answering this question is often used as an argument against virtue theory itself, as Veatch is doing in the article just cited. But this is a particularly weak objection against this form of virtue theory, since it leaves virtue theory no worse off than its competitors. Just as with principles or paradigm cases, for example, virtues may be inherited in the core of a settled morality; or they may be indexed to a foundational goal (as Aristotle's virtues were taken to serve human happiness); or they may be tested by their fit within a reflective equilibrium of virtues, principles, and considered judgments.

There's no reason, then, to think that arguments on behalf of particular virtues, or their interpretations or applications, won't encounter the same sorts of limits discussed in other chapters of this book. We'll encounter some examples of this later.

What Does "*Virtue*" Require?

A second question is whether virtues as moral excellences require only the disposition to act rightly. Being a "respectful" physician would then mean nothing but being a person who habitually listens to patients' stories, takes account of their values, refrains from saying disparaging things to or about them, and so on. But this would make attribution of the virtue a shorthand way of praising the action, not also the actor. What's needed is an acknowledgment that people can do the right things for less than the best reasons. A physician might scrupulously get his patients' informed consent because he fears his legal liability if he doesn't. He's doing the right thing, but his doing of it reflects no moral credit on him. So possessing a virtue requires more that conforming one's action to a rule, even the rule that might seem constitutive of the virtue.

This might lead us to think that the possession of virtue requires only that one be well motivated. This can't be right either, because it would imply, for example, that trying to be compassionate is all it takes to be a compassionate person. To the contrary, no matter how earnest I am, if I'm always putting my foot in my mouth in ways that inadvertently hurt others, or I often misgauge the needs of those I wish to help, then I've failed to be a compassionate person; not because of ill will, but because of incompetence.

Thus, both the disposition and the capacity to act rightly are only necessary, but not sufficient, conditions for the possession of virtues; what that possession requires in addition is a set of laudable, rather than base, motives for acting. The language of virtues and vices is a language for the appraisal of those motives, and of the persons who act from them. Importantly, this language of virtue depends on our *independent* ability to characterize the rightness or wrongness of acts, for this is how we judge whether a person has the capacity to act in accordance with the virtue. To be a fair person requires not just that I act from a desire to be fair, but that what I do is in fact fair. Both myself and others must be able to ascertain that fact before the virtue of fairness can properly be attributed to me. This means, as Hursthouse points out, that a virtue theory concerned with the moral excellence of persons cannot be a reductionist one, "defining all our moral concepts in terms of the virtues" (Hursthouse, 1997, p. 221).

In What Way is *"Virtue"* a Supplementary Language?

The virtues and vices, then, offer a supplementary, not an alternative, ethical language. But now another question arises. In what way is this language supplementary? Is it merely that where before we had only a language for appraising actions, we've now added a language for appraising persons? Or have we also in some way added to the language we have available for appraising actions themselves? The answer will affect how we explain the relevance of virtue for health care ethics.

Suppose first that virtues and vices make up a separate language that appraises persons but not their acts. The challenge is to explain why this should matter to our practical concerns in modern health care ethics. Robert Veatch remarks, "I think it can be reasonably said that in the world of strangers, we are much more concerned about conduct then [sic] virtuous character. If we could be assured that the physician would do the right thing, we would not really be concerned about motivation" (Veatch, 1985, p. 339). Perhaps in a bygone age, when the doctor was our neighbor and friend, we might have had some concern for the well-being of his soul. But when the doctor is someone unknown to us, what matters is only *that* he's treated us right, not *why* he did so.

This misses the mark in several directions. First, it makes the implausible assumption that one could easily establish systems of reward and punishment that could replace good intentions as a guarantor of good behavior. To the contrary, we should care about physicians' characters if only because we care about their behavior. Seeing to the former is a primary, and probably irreplaceable, way of encouraging the latter. If my physician is following my wishes only out of fear of getting her hand slapped for doing otherwise, I have reason to be apprehensive. I'll always be subject to the vagaries in her calculations of the risk of getting caught.

The second problem is the implicit argument that because the patient might not much care about his doctor's character, the discipline of health care ethics shouldn't care either. This presupposes that patients and their needs are the only legitimate objects of moral concern. Surely, however, the professional character of practitioners is part of the moral universe encompassed by a professional ethics. Even if no one but professionals cared about it, it would still be a proper object for study, education, and training.

The third, and most important, problem with an argument like Veatch's is just the assumption that the virtues and vices are always irrelevant to the evaluation of actions (and for this reason of no interest to the patient affected by only what the physician *does*).

But the boundary between the assessment of persons and the assessment of their acts is not always clear. Take the physician's obligation to treat the patient "with respect." To act respectfully requires not only certain behaviors, but certain motives as well. If my doctor is acting just as nice as can be, but all the while fuming inside over what an idiot I am, then his action can no longer be described as "respectful." At best, he's only being "polite." If as his patient I want him to treat me "with respect," I will be interested not only in his behavior, but in his motives as well.

Better knowledge of his motives, beliefs, and commitments might lead me to describe his treatment of me as "grudging" or "cynical" or "dishonest." Such moral characterizations of his actions are inseparable from a characterization of him and his motives.

Hursthouse illustrates in her discussion of abortion how such a virtue perspective can open up new and fruitful avenues for moral reflection and criticism. Even if we think that a woman has a moral right to choose an abortion, she may make that choice in a shallow, hasty, selfish, or callous way. Even if we allow that the ultimate moral status of the fetus—whether it has a right to life—is contested and radically unsettled, we may still argue that certain attitudes toward it are less admirable than others. For Hursthouse, the evaluation of these attitudes is indexed to certain other values she takes to be inherent in the facts of human social life—for example, that parents do, and should, feel love for their children; that being a parent adds meaning and fulfillment to one's life (although it's not the only way to do so). Woman (and, equally, the men in their lives) may act from motives that deny values such as these. A person who chooses abortion thinking the fetus is just a lump of flesh like a tumor betrays a callousness that is oblivious to the fetus' developmental and symbolic connection to beloved children. This callousness in us would be strikingly revealed, for example, were we to remark to a woman who is grieving a miscarriage that she should think of it as nothing more than a heavy period.

The added dimensions of moral evaluation that motives can offer should not lead us to exaggerate their role. Motive is not, Peter Abelard to the contrary[6], the sole source of moral value. Again, Hursthouse's discussion is instructive. Even if a woman has made a choice for abortion hastily, it may still properly be her right to have one; it may still be the best choice for her circumstances; it may still be the choice that best meets the legitimate interests of others, including the fetus; and so on. Of course, one might say that if her choice were deficient in any of these other ways, it would also lack "virtue;" and that a choice that's deficient

in none of these ways epitomizes "virtue." Used this way, however, "virtue" has become just another omnibus term of moral
approval, synonymous with "right," "good," and the like. The
phrase "virtue ethics" would be a redundancy, "virtue" marking
nothing distinctive about the ethics being practiced.

Some Appeals to Virtue in Medical Ethics

Consideration of some of the ways that virtue has appeared
in medical ethics will illustrate some of these points, and
suggest in more concrete ways the uses and limits of appeals to
virtues.

The Doctrine of Double Effect

The Doctrine of Double Effect (DDE) has been used extensively
in medical ethics. Although stated as a principle, what is significant about it for our present discussion is that it appeals to intention or motive to mark the boundary between the permissible
and the impermissible. It is in that respect an application of a
virtue ethic.

The DDE has a long history in Jewish and Roman Catholic
moral theology, and that history has seen a variety of formula-
tions of the doctrine.[7] Although the differences between these
can significantly affect the application of the doctrine, for my
purposes I will use what is perhaps the most common formulation: It is permissible to perform an action that has both a good
and a bad effect so long as:

1. The act in itself is not evil or impermissible.
2. The good effect, and not the bad one, is the effect intended
   (even though the bad effect is a foreseen consequence).

3. The bad effect is not the means used for achieving the good effect.
4. There is a proportionately grave reason for permitting the bad effect (e.g., the good effect outweighs the bad effect).

The heart of the doctrine is the second condition. The first and the last conditions set moral boundaries that are independent of the agent's intentions, ensuring that the act is not objectionable on deontological or utilitarian grounds. The third condition is merely a criterion for assessing whether the bad effect is not also intended, employing the idea that one cannot intend the effect without also intending the means.

The distinction between intended and merely foreseen consequences has most often been used in medical ethics to identify those deaths for which the physician is not morally culpable. One application concerns the use of pain medication. The physician who administers morphine in doses large enough to hasten her patient's death is not culpable so long as the intention was to relieve pain and not to bring about a quicker death (e.g., Pellegrino, 1998; Schneiderman and Spragg, 1988). Another application draws a distinction between "active" and "passive" euthanasia. It may be permissible to withdraw a life-sustaining treatment such as a ventilator, even knowing death will certainly result, but it's never permissible to achieve the same result by administering a lethal injection. In the first instance, the physician's intention may be to relieve the patient of the burden of treatment, rather than bring about the patient's death; whereas in the second instance death must be among the intentions (e.g., see Sullivan, 1977). It is with respect to intentions that some argue that the withdrawal of treatment can be ethically tantamount to euthanasia—withdrawing artificial food and fluids from a patient in a persistent vegetative state, for example, can have no plausible purpose other than bringing about the patient's death (see Meilaender, 1984).

Most criticism of such applications of DDE focuses on the difficulty in discerning what the actor's intentions in fact are, or on the problems encountered in explaining how an effect can be foreseen, and accepted, but not intended. These are pertinent criticisms of the doctrine, but they don't go directly to its emphasis on the character of the agent as the basis on which the act is to be judged. In this regard, there are two more fundamental questions to be asked about such uses of the DDE. First, why should such an intention, even if thought to be wrong, alone be sufficient to make the action itself wrong? Second, why should we think that such an intention is always wrong?

The first question relates to the point made earlier—that acts done from bad motives may in all other respects be defensible, and for that reason *permissible*, even if not *admirable*. Why mightn't that be the case here? Imagine two conscious, competent, respirator-dependent patients with COPD who wish the ventilator withdrawn. The one can no longer tolerate the discomfort and restrictions caused by the machine, but would be pleased if a miracle occurred and he survived the withdrawal, even with the severe disability that would remain. The other feels the same way about the machine, but is counting on not surviving the withdrawal, because he can no longer bear the disabilities of his illness. Why should the one be thought ethically permissible, and the other not? Each act is equally in accord with the patient's rights and interests. Each act has the same foreseeable consequence—the patient dies. If one insists that the second patient is doing the right thing for the wrong reason, he's nevertheless still doing the right thing, as judged by every other ethical criterion. If he's still open to moral criticism, it will not be so much for the choice that he makes, but for his reason for that choice. We might say it is his *choosing* that is suspect, not his *choice*.

When a supposedly wrongful motive operates independently of the other moral features of choices, it's hard to see how the motive by itself is grounds for condemning a choice that would otherwise be permissible. Motives are most plausibly relevant when they have an effect on these other features.[8] So, in the present context, one has more relevant grounds for distinguishing between active and passive euthanasia on the basis of motive if one can successfully argue that the motive behind the former is more subject to insidious distortions that lead, for example, to non-voluntary killing.

Such implications of motives not only make them more relevant to questions of policy; they are the basis on which the motive is claimed to be a "vicious" rather than a virtuous one. Why is it reprehensible to be the sort of physician who would agree to kill the innocent patient, when she has made a free and informed request? One might argue, like Leon Kass (1991) does, that such an act is incompatible with the integrity of medicine and the integrity of the good physician. Why? Perhaps because it is at odds with medicine's Hippocratic tradition, which specifically prohibits "giving poison." Perhaps because it is incompatible with the essential goal of healing (Kass, 1991). But now one must be prepared to defend one's selective reliance on the Hippocratic tradition (which also forbade surgery); and one must be prepared to defend the idea that healing is the only, or is the absolute, goal that medicine might have (see Momeyer, 1995).

In either case, our condemnation of the motive behind physician-assisted death, and of the acts that proceed from it, must rely on reasons that look beyond virtue, and depend on claims about the proper source of moral authority in medicine, the proper goals of the profession, the likely consequences of acting from such motives, and so on. In these ways, the arguments made within a "virtue ethics" will look remarkably like the arguments found within a "rule ethics."

Refusal to Treat AIDS Patients

Another example is found in the debate from the early days of the AIDS epidemic: Do physicians have an individual obligation to provide care to patients with HIV/AIDS within their area of competence, despite the very small risk of infection they would run? As John Arras (1988) pointed out, appeals to principles had the effect of locating the obligation to treat in the profession as a whole, rather than in each individual physician. If patients with AIDS have a right to care, that right can be met so long as the profession sees to it that someone competent is available to provide it. If the social contract, by means of which physicians enjoy monopoly power, in turn obligates them to meet the health care needs of society's vulnerable members, that is as well an obligation that can be discharged by the profession as a whole, without imposing it on every member. Of course, one might respond to such attempted deflections of duty with pragmatic arguments maintaining that the only practical way the profession is going to discharge its duties is by enforcing an obligation on all of its members individually. Indeed, Arras does just that. But this is a dissatisfying strategy, he admits. The resulting duty is a merely instrumental one, and the failure to discharge it only the reluctance to play one's small part in the larger enterprise.

The duty to treat is therefore a question that begs to be addressed from the perspective of professional virtue. Only if understood as an expression of that virtue will the duty be one equally binding on all physicians individually. But how can the requirement for such a virtue be established? Arras considers several forms of argument. One is drawn from Zuger and Miles, and argues that the profession's defining commitment to the goal of healing entails an altruistic commitment to care for those in need. This is essentially an argument from principle, and it is prey to all the familiar sorts of challenges. There is the matter of its interpretation, for example, for a physician might profess a commitment to care for the ill, but insist that this virtue is expressed in the sacrifices he makes for those who are already his patients. It doesn't require that he care for all comers. There is also the now-familiar problem of assessing the weight of this virtue against that of other virtues and duties with which it might be in tension. A physician might properly feel love and concern for the welfare of her family, which would lead her to consider the risk they might be exposed to (directly or indirectly) were the physician to contract HIV/AIDS. Unless the virtue of altruism is absolute, there must be some permissible level of risk avoidance in order to accommodate the expression of other virtues and duties. But this principled form of argument won't tell us where that level lies.

These problems lead Arras to embrace another strategy, which is to argue that the virtue of self-sacrifice, with its willingness to take risks to help the sick, is embedded in the moral tradition of the profession. A major difficulty here is with the factual premise. Does the profession's history unambiguously express such a virtue? Arras spends much of his time struggling with the complexity of the historical record. The more fundamental problem, however, is to explain why the virtues of the profession should be established by its history. One difficulty with any stark reliance on history is that it offers no reason why the historical tradition should continue. After all, there's much in the tradition we're glad to be rid of. The facts of history won't sort the wheat from the chaff. The other is that "tradition" is a matter of what the profession actually does or endorses, and that is subject to change. Arras bemoans evidence (circa 1988) showing the extent to which younger physicians claim a right not to treat AIDS patients. If that attitude were to become the norm, a new tradition will have emerged that offered no grounds for complaint. (Indeed, there are still substantial minorities of physician who are reluctant to provide care to patients with HIV/AIDS; see Frater, 1999.)

There is finally a third strategy, to which Arras pays the least attention, but which may be a mode of argument distinctive of a virtue ethics. It is to link the duty to treat to other, more central virtues. So, for example, Arras suggests that the physician who shrinks from treating AIDS patients betrays a lack of empathy, understood as a spontaneous responsiveness to those in need. This is a quality of mind we want all physicians to have, but spontaneous responsiveness is incompatible with careful calculation of self-interest. The incompatibility is not a matter of inconsistency within a set of rules, or other logical system, or a matter of what it means to "be empathetic." Being empathetic does not require one never to calculate self-interest, or never to refuse any patient. The concern is not with this or that particular incident. It's with a habit of mind. The incompatibility is a matter of moral psychology: the physician who calculates his risk exposure with every patient undermines his ability to respond empathetically to their needs. This is not a conceptual claim or a moral claim. It's an empirical one that would need the support of psychological evidence, not philosophical argument.

Whatever the fate of this particular argument, it illustrates a mode of reasoning that is of particular importance for a virtue ethics. Without it, our virtue ethics is likely to be pretty unilluminating. To say that physicians should have the virtue of truthfulness because they have a duty to tell the truth to their patients tells us little about either the virtue or the duty. To say that physicians should have the virtue of compassion because they should be able to act in ways that are sensitive to the needs of their patients is equally unhelpful. We need to know what other traits of character help or hinder the capacity to tell the truth when it's called for. Perhaps humility is a psychological prerequisite for admitting a medical mistake, for example (Andre, 2000).

We need to know what patterns of behavior, what kinds of habitual choices, what working and learning environments lead to cynicism, loathing, and the withering of compassion among physicians (e.g., see Coulehan and Williams, 2001). Only with such mappings of the connections between attitudes, behaviors, choice, and environments will we be able to say anything very sophisticated about what particular virtues the ethical practice of medicine really requires, about what particular choices are incompatible with those virtues, or about how we can best foster and protect the virtuous physician.

Conclusion

A virtue ethics cannot substitute for, or operate independently of, other forms of moral knowledge, including moral principles. Virtues like prudence are not usefully thought of as unique epistemic powers of moral perception. Nevertheless, virtue can offer a fresh perspective, not only regarding the character of individual physicians, but regarding their choices as well. Often, the sorts of considerations offered in support claims about particular virtues or their implications for particular choices are similar in character to those used in other forms of moral argument. But a full understanding of the medical virtues requires a sophisticated moral psychology, not just philosophical analysis.

Notes

1. Note that we need to ask the same question about ourselves, and so it gets us nowhere to say that the virtuous person knows that whatever she chooses is the right thing to do. What warrants her confidence in her own virtue?

2. E.g., see the issue of *Theoretical Medicine* edited by Tomlinson (1986).

3. And so Rosalind Hursthouse admits that on her account of virtue theory, in such circumstances neither party can claim that the other is wrong (Hursthouse, 1997, note 1, p. 219).

4. In his article, Kihlbom is defending care theory, as a kind of virtue theory, against the objections brought by Helga Kuhse. This is the same nurse I discussed in my chapter on feminist approaches.

5. By the end of his article, Kihlbom is endorsing a coherence model of justification: "A particular moral view can be criticized for not cohering with our more general moral views, and vice versa" (Kihlbom, 2000, p. 309).

6. See McInerny's discussion of Abelard in the *Encyclopedia of Ethics* (1992, pp. 1–2).

7. See the useful discussion by Marquis (1991).

8. Of course, we do distinguish between accidental and deliberate killing. Genuine accidents aren't objects of moral condemnation; deliberate killings often are. But this is not because accidental killings are done from good motives. They're not done from any motive at all— that is, they are not products of deliberation or the lack of it. They fall outside the realm of moral responsibility altogether.

Bibliography

Andre, Judith. 2000. "Humility Reconsidered." In *Margin of Error: The Ethics of Mistakes in the Practice of Medicine*. Ed. Susan B. Rubin and Laurie Zoloth. Hagerstown: University Publishing Group, pp. 59–72.

Aristotle. 1941. "Nicomachean Ethics." In *The Basic Works of Aristotle*, ed. Richard McKeon. New York: Random House.

Arras, John D. 1988. "The Fragile Web of Responsibility: AIDS and the Duty to Treat." *Hastings Center Report* (April-May), pp. 10–19.

Coulehan, Jack and Peter C. Williams. 2001. "Vanquishing Virtue: The Impact of Medical Education." *Academic Medicine* 76(6): 598–605.

Frater, R. W. 1999. As originally published in 1989: human immunodeficiency virus and the cardiac surgeon: a survey of attitudes. Updated in 1999. *Annals of Thoracic Surgery* 67(4):1203–1204.

Hursthouse, Rosalind. 1997. "Virtue Theory and Abortion." In *Virtue Ethics*, ed. Roger Crisp and Michael Slote. Oxford: Oxford University Press.

Jansen, Lynn A. 2000. "The Virtues in their Place: Virtue Ethics in Medicine." *Theoretical Medicine* 21: 261–276.

Kass, Leon R. 1991. "Why Doctors Must Not Kill." *Commonweal* 118(14):472–476.

Katz, Jay. 1984. *The Silent World of Doctor and Patient*. New York: The Free Press.

Kihlbom, Ulrik. 2000. "Guidance and Justification in Particularistic Ethics." *Bioethics* 14 (4): 287–309.

Lo, Bernard. 1988. "Obligations to Care for Persons with Human Immunodeficiency Virus." *Issues in Law and Medicine* 4(3): 367–381.

Louden, Robert B. 1984. "On Some Vices of Virtue Ethics." *American Philosophical Quarterly* 21(3):227–236.

Marquis, Donald B. 1991. "Four Versions of Double Effect." *Journal of Medicine and Philosophy* 16:515–544.

McDowell, John. 1989. "Virtue and Reason." In *Anti-Theory in Ethics and Moral Conservatism*, ed. Stanley G. Clarke and Evan Simpson. State University of New York Press.

McInerny, Ralph. 1992. "Peter Abelard." *Encyclopedia of Ethics*. Ed. L. C. Becker and C. B. Becker. New York: Garland, pp. 1–2.

MacIntyre, Alasdair. 1984. *After Virtue*, 2nd ed. Notre Dame, IN: Notre Dame Press.

Meilaender, Gilbert. 1984. "On Removing Food and Water: Against the Stream." *Hastings Center Report* Dec., pp. 11–13.

Momeyer, Richard. 1995. "Does Physician-Assisted Suicide Violate the Integrity of Medicine?" *Journal of Medicine and Philosophy* 20(1): 13–24.

Nussbaum, Martha C. 1999. "Virtue Ethics: A Misleading Category." *Journal of Ethics* 3:163–201.

Pellegrino, Edmund D. 1995. "Toward a Virtue-Based Normative Ethics for the Health Professions." *Kennedy Institute of Ethics Journal* 5(3):253–277.

Pellegrino, Edmund D. 1998. "Emerging Ethical Issues in Palliative Care." *Journal of the American Medical Association* 279:1521–1522.

Pellegrino, Edmund D. and David C. Thomasma. 1993. *The Virtues in Medical Practice*. New York: Oxford University Press.

Rothman, David J. 1991. *Strangers at the Bedside: A History of How Law and Bioethics Transformed Medical Decision-making*. Basic Books.

Schneewind, J. B. 1990. "The Misfortunes of Virtue." *Ethics* 101 (October), pp. 42–63.

Schneiderman, Lawrence J. and Roger G. Spragg. 1988. "Ethical Decisions in Discontinuing Mechanical Ventilation." *New England Journal of Medicine* 318:984–988.

Sullivan, Thomas D. 1977. "Active and Passive Euthanasia: An Impertinent Distinction?" *Human Life Review* 3(3):40–46. Reprinted in Thomas A. Mappes and Jane Zembaty, eds. 1986. *Biomedical Ethics*. New York: McGraw-Hill, pp. 388–392.

Tomlinson, Tom. Ed. 1986. "The Physician's Influence on Patient Decision-making: Persuasion, Manipulation, and Coercion." *Theoretical Medicine*, June.

Veatch, Robert M. 1985. "Against Virtue: A Deontological Critique of Virtue Theory in Medical Ethics. In *Virtue and Medicine*, ed. Earl E. Shelp. Dordrecht: Reidel.

Zuger, Abrigail and Miles, Steven. 1987. "Physicians, AIDS, and occupational risk. Historic traditions and ethical obligations." *Journal of the American Medical Association*. 258(14):1924–8.

Chapter 8

Fitting Methods to Cases

In the book I've characterized a variety of methods, and identified some of their strengths and weaknesses. It would be tempting at this stage to rank order them with regard to their global adequacy or usefulness. This would assume, however, that we not only have some plausible metric for "usefulness," but that the ethical questions we confront differ not at all in the sorts of tools required for their analysis or resolution. Do different sorts of problems yield to different sorts of tools? Do different tools play distinctive roles in the analysis and resolution of ethical questions? I will pursue these questions in this chapter.

Types of Ethical Tools

It will be helpful to further characterize the roles methods can play under two headings: tools for ethical discovery, and tools for ethical justification.

A **tool for ethical discovery** is a method or perspective that helps us uncover ethically salient features of a situation that enrich our understanding of the nature of the ethical problem or question. I don't mean to refer simply to any deliberate collection of ethically relevant facts. I may, for example, conduct an empirical study to determine whether surrogate decision-makers accurately represent the values and preferences of patients (Tomlinson, Howe, Notman, and Mitchell, 1990). The object is to determine whether a certain ideal of substituted judgment is being met. The facts will tell me to what degree it is or is not. Although it may prompt me to further investigation, the answer leaves my beginning assumption intact—that the patient's values and preferences are the only ethical feature of interest. The results (especially if they are disappointing) may motivate me to reconsider my beginning assumption, but by themselves they don't broaden my ethical vision of what is at stake in these situations.

To do that, I might instead ask patients to explain why they executed an advance directive, what process of thought or discussion led up to it, and so on. Or I might ask families to explain how they made decisions about the care of an incapacitated loved one. I might, in other words, gather a number of *stories* concerning patient and family decision-making about end-of-life care. This more open-ended inquiry could yield not just new factual information, but new information about the values that must be accounted for in any further ethical analysis (e.g., see High, 1988).

Several of the methods we have discussed offer tools of ethical discovery in this sense. Narrative methods are one example, of course, through the eliciting of stories or "counterstories." (Also see Tovey's [1998] discussion of the uses of "life stories" as a tool of empirical ethics.) Casuistry is another, in particular through the use of paradigm cases to identify additional relevant ethical features that bear investigation. Within feminist ethics, standpoint theory can also serve as a tool of discovery.

Notably, principle-centered methods, including wide reflective equilibrium, do not offer tools of ethical discovery, except by the minimal way of providing an ethical vocabulary that frames the investigation of an ethical difficulty. The application of these methods assumes that we've already fully characterized the ethical situation, accounting for all the values at stake. Principle-centered methods are instead the paradigm example of a **tool of ethical justification**. Tools of ethical justification are used to construct or to evaluate a set of reasons offered in support of a moral conclusion. They do so by employing some standard by which actions or states of affairs are to be judged better or worse, right or wrong. On this account, casuistry also aspires to be a tool of ethical justification, judging actions by their relation to paradigm cases. So too is a virtue theory that judges the desirability of traits by reference to some overarching goal. A feminist analysis may also justify moral criticism of a particular practice, when it demonstrates how the practice unfairly affects women. Narrative ethics aims to offer a tool of ethical justification when it proposes narrative coherence as a benchmark for moral rightness.

In any particular instance of its use, a method can fail as a tool of ethical justification yet still succeed as a tool of ethical discovery, as we saw in our discussions of narrative ethics and casuistry. And discovery can lead to a warranted ethical conclusion, even if it's not the method of discovery that warrants it. When the elicitation of further stories reveals ethical considerations that decisively tip the balance in favor of one course of action, that discovery has also served to provide reasons in favor of that conclusion. When a casuistical investigation shows decisively that the case under consideration is an instance of a paradigm case, we know what to do without further argument.

As we discuss different types of ethical problems below, a method may sometimes be useful as a tool of justification, a tool of discovery, or both.

Types of Ethical Problems

At considerable risk of over-simplifying, I plan to discuss uses for the methods we've discussed in three different types of ethical problem:

1. Decisions about what to do in a specific, concrete case or situation
2. Decisions about whether to endorse a statement of ethical principle, ideal, or virtue
3. Decisions about the desirability of a practice, policy, or law

These are obviously not mutually exclusive sorts of problems, but can intersect in a variety of ways. A decision about a case may turn on the acceptance of a key principle, and it may be generalized to support a recommendation for policy. Still, I hope to show that the argumentative demands differ significantly across these three types in ways that affect the usefulness of methods.

Decisions About Cases

A decision about what to do in a specific case has a number of features that may affect the usefulness of a method. First, it requires that we be knowledgeable about all of the ethically pertinent facts, which will be facts about that particular state of affairs. It will require that we place those facts within some larger ethical framework (or frameworks) that provides the ethical valences for the various factors present, explaining why each of these favors one course of action or another. And we will then need to make some evaluation of the cogency and weight of the strands of reasons we've assembled, and make a decision about where the ethical evidence points.

I will use a case and commentary from the *Journal of Clinical Ethics* (2002) to illustrate how the various methods we've discussed could help answer such questions. Through a series of interviews and reports by various parties, "Irene's Story" describes the situation of a middle-aged Russian immigrant seeking to have a third child. Previous attempts to conceive by use of both AID and IVF with donor sperm failed due to a diminished number of eggs in her ovaries. The option of using both donor eggs and sperm was offered, and she elected to pursue it. She insisted, however, that her father be the sperm donor. Her father, who lived with her and helped care for his two grandchildren, supported the idea, and agreed to the collection of several vials of viable sperm. This had to be done by testicular biopsy; because he'd had a prostatectomy, he was unable to ejaculate. The patient revealed this plan to the infertility center's social worker during a standard interview. The social worker, concerned about a number of issues, referred the case for review by the Egg Donor Committee, which acts as a *de facto* ethics committee for the Center. In the end, the Committee decided to deny Irene's request.[1] How might this decision be defended, and how could the reasons supporting it be evaluated?

The most obvious first step in this exploration would be to ask the various protagonists to explain their points of view. Many of these—although not all—will be shot through with explicit or implicit appeals to moral principles or rules. This was the case here. The social worker refers to the National Association of Social Workers' Code of Ethics, and its injunction that "Social workers may limit clients' right to self-determination when, in the social workers' professional judgment, clients' actions or potential actions pose a serious, foreseeable, and imminent risk to themselves or others" (O'Neill, 2002, p. 233). For her part, Irene asserts that "Since Hippocratic times, the patient has been proclaimed the main and unique object of medicine. As such, ethics needs to first consider the patient's needs." In her commentary, Klipstein (2002c) claims the main question is whether Irene's plan would violate the rule against incest.

For the reasons discussed earlier, such invocations of principles are virtually unavoidable. Ethical stances, particularly in cases of disagreement, demand reasons, and principles are a prominent form of reason. In addition, some framework of general convictions is necessary for identifying those elements of the situation that are morally salient. However, in this case as elsewhere, principles alone may underdetermine any single conclusion. Even if the social worker makes a case that there is some risk (e.g., for "role confusion") created by Irene's plans, there will still be the question of whether this risk is "serious" or "imminent" or unavoidable enough to justify not respecting the decision that Irene and her father have made. For reasons discussed in earlier chapters, this balancing judgment cannot be warranted by appeal to some further principle. If there is any more reasoned reflection possible, it will be by some other means.

One of those other means is to critically examine the arguments and evidence offered for the competing considerations. This critical examination aims either to undermine the import of a well-grounded principle for the particular case or to demonstrate that a principle being invoked is not itself well grounded. These are both ways to alter the balance of moral considerations enough to clearly warrant one conclusion rather than another.

Both Klipstein (2002c) and Forrow (2002b) adopt the first strategy in their commentaries, which are both skeptical of the social worker's position. The social worker claims that the child might suffer role and identity confusions—his father is also his grandfather, and his mother is also his half-sister. She worries that he might be stigmatized by his unusual origins. She is also concerned that the father's participation might not be entirely voluntary, since he is financially and socially dependent on his daughter, and so potentially subject to manipulation. But Klipstein contends that concern over harm to the child caused by role confusions assumes that the child must be told who his biological father is. It also assumes that the grandfather will unavoidably be cast into playing the social role of father as well. Even if the beans are spilled, Klipstein asserts that it is entirely speculative to insist that the child will be seriously or unavoidably harmed by any stigma. Regarding the voluntariness of the father's participation, Forrow points out that since no effort was made to speak with Irene's father, no one was in a position to claim that his participation was anything but completely voluntary.

The intended effect of these counter-arguments is to undermine the credibility of the social worker's claims that Irene's plans in fact threaten the interests or rights of others, and in doing so they try to shift the weight of evidence. If successful, they shift the weight enough to favor allowing Irene's choice. As discussed earlier, there are no decisive criteria for judging that this tipping point has been reached. It will be sufficient if the arguments lead to a consensus about which course of action the reasons favor, a consensus based in a common moral sensibility.

So one way to undermine the import of a principle is to question specific background factual assumptions linking it to the situation. Another is to argue that a well-grounded principle is being misinterpreted in its application to the case. This sort of argument can be casuistical. Is Irene proposing to engage in some kind of "incest," as the social worker suggests? Irene herself points to disanalogies with the typical "incest" subject to prohibition. The conception of her child will not be the result of intercourse, nor will it even involve the union of her father's sperm with her eggs. Klipstein also compares what Irene proposes with several different varieties of "incest," and finds what she takes to be significant differences. She notes, however, that one of the "most disturbing aspects [of Irene's proposal] may be that Irene would, in essence, be carrying her father's child and her own half-sibling" (Klipstein, 2002c, p. 241). Although she doesn't further explain what is disturbing about this, the implication is that the hint of incest remains even after its more unsettling elements have been subtracted from our judgment. The question will be whether this lingering moral residue should be enough for us not to cooperate in Irene's plans. It's possible that a common moral sensibility will produce an unproblematic answer to the question. An alternative looks for the answer in a paradigmatic case, or what's taken to be one. This is the avenue chosen by several of the commentators, who point out that the clinic has a policy that permits brother–sister gamete donation, around which the same faint whiff of incest lingers. Of course, this might not end the matter, if there are those prepared to claim that there are morally unique elements to the father–daughter relation that justify treating it differently for these purposes.

Finally, instead of shifting the balance of argument by challenging the relevance of a principle to the situation, one might instead challenge the cogency of one of the principles being invoked. Although none of the commentators did this, one might well question the idea that Irene has a right of autonomy that creates a *prima facie* obligation for the clinic to respect her decision. Someone might argue that this claim is poorly connected to our more settled considered judgments regarding the right of autonomy. Most of these concern the right not to be interfered with; Irene is asking not just to be left alone, but to be assisted by others. This appeal to the standard distinction between positive and negative rights would only be the first salvo in an argument claiming that an interpretation of the right of autonomy that compels the clinic's cooperation is not well grounded within a wide reflective equilibrium.

So far we have seen how appeals to principles will naturally arise in any discussion of an ethically difficult case. As we should expect, these will lead to the need to balance competing principles, and interpret their meaning and relevance in the particular context of the case. A careful understanding of the facts can help in our assessment of the weight of evidence behind the alternatives proposed. The method of wide reflective equilibrium may be used to test the cogency of key principles. Paradigm cases and casuistical reasoning may help us judge whether principles are being properly interpreted in their application to the case.

What of the other methods discussed in this book? Narrative certainly may have a role to play in this case. In the interview with her, Irene explains her decision to have a third child in middle age by saying that it would prevent her family from "dwindling," the fate of many families in Russia at the time. This is the start of a story that is not further drawn out by the interviewer, and none of the commentators makes anything of it. But one can readily imagine from this hint that for Irene this child has special significance in a struggle to continue a cultural and ethnic legacy that is in danger of disappearing. Within this story, her desire to use her father as the sperm donor takes on a new meaning, since his donation ensures that the child will be at least part Russian, and continues a familial blood line. Such a story has three possible uses. The first is to introduce a new moral question: is such a transpersonal project one to which the fertility center should give its allegiance? A second is to suggest an account of Irene's motives that further distances them from charges of incest. In the first, the narrative has served as a tool of ethical discovery, by revealing an ethical consideration not before apparent. In the second, the narrative has added to our understanding of the facts in a way that might tip the balance of ethical argument in favor of honoring her request. Finally, the story suggests an alternative course of action that might offer a resolution to the ethical conflict between Irene and the Center: finding a Russian sperm donor other than her father.

A feminist analysis might also be useful here, in particular to understand any ways in which Irene's apparently autonomous choice may be constrained by unarticulated and unchallenged assumptions regarding a woman's—particularly a Russian woman's—proper role. As we saw in our discussion of feminist methods, it is dangerous to rely on generalizations regarding classes of women. Any such analysis would have to depend on a much better understanding of Irene's character and history, supplied by a richer narrative of her life than the case history provides. Although also not apparent in the case history, a richer narrative might reveal as well questionable motives that would alter our assessment of the moral character of Irene's decisions. But given what we have, these are only speculations.

As our discussion of Irene's case has illustrated, the whole array of methods we've discussed may find some use in making judgments about particular cases. This is not to say that each method will find a use in every case. Perhaps, for example, the case lies too far outside the boundaries of settled paradigmatic cases to give casuistical methods any foothold. Or the array of ethical principles and moral considerations brought to bear are in themselves decisive enough that they don't require any adjudication by means of wide reflective equilibrium.

Perhaps more importantly, we need to notice that the methods employed got used for different purposes. The organizing structure for the debate was provided by a set of principles—regarding the prohibition of incest, the obligation to avoid harming the child to be conceived, the obligation to respect autonomous decisions, and so on. The overarching question was how to weight the relevance and significance of these for a decision about the case. Some of the other methods were then useful for answering this question. Casuistry proved helpful in determining whether the prohibition against incest sensibly applied to these circumstances, for example. Other methods—like narrative—promised more by way of ethical discovery, uncovering further details that could inform interpretations of the principles under contention. What this suggests is that these other methods are ancillary to the use of principles, useful insofar as they can be put in the service of deciding what conclusions the principles can warrant. It's not that non-principle methods are less important in ethical reflection. Indeed, they may often decide the argument. Rather, they are useful and important precisely when they can affect the interpretation and cogency of principle-based ethical argument.

Decisions About Principles

A second aspect of ethical judgment is deciding what attitude to take to a statement of moral principle, virtue, or ideal. "It's wrong for a doctor to kill, even with the patient's consent." "Patients should understand as much as possible about their medical condition." Claims such as these play critical roles in explaining more particular judgments, as we've just seen. They also invite several sorts of questions. How should the principle, and the key concepts used in it, be understood? How do different understandings affect its scope, the variety of acts it permits or prohibits? Under which of its interpretations, if any, is the principle true; and for what reasons?

How can the methods we've canvassed in this book help answer these questions? Let's take as our illustrative example the claim that a physician has a right to refuse to provide futile care demanded by a patient or family.

I have written on this issue quite a bit, and tend to cautiously favor the claim that physicians have such a prerogative (Tomlinson and Brody, 1990 Tomlinson, 2001, 2007; Tomlinson and Czlonka, 1995). In my discussion here I won't argue for any particular substantive view on the matter, but instead will focus on strategies to address it, and how they employ the various methods we've explored.

Since the claim asserts a general ethical principle, it is not surprising if the evaluation of it will require some appeal to other ethical principles. This starts with the apparent conflict that has made the claim a contentious one for twenty years. On the one hand, patients (and the families or others acting in their name) are seen to have a right of autonomy regarding their medical treatment. Isn't it a violation of that right for a physician to deny the treatment autonomously demanded by the patient? But then on the other hand, physicians can cause harm to patients by what they do and should only be recommending interventions that have some prospect of benefit—a basic norm of professional integrity. Isn't it a violation of professional integrity, then, for physicians to provide useless and even harmful "treatments," even when patients demand them?

So principles will establish the framework that structures the problem, and that will determine the broad strategies for evaluating the claim. To evaluate the claim, we will need to evaluate both the soundness of each of the competing principles, and the application of those principles to the context of decisions about treatment.

Some of this evaluation could appeal to yet other principles, perhaps grounded in widely acknowledged paradigm cases. For example, one might ask why refusing to provide a treatment the patient demands is a violation of her right of autonomy. In the medical context, the right of patient autonomy is most commonly understood as the right to refuse treatment, a right recognized by the courts in many individual cases. But the right to refuse treatment is a right to bodily integrity, to non-interference, one might say. Understood this way, there is no violation of the patient's right to autonomy when the physician *refuses to do* something to the patient, rather than *insists on doing* something to the patient. And so, if there is anything wrong with the physician refusing a demand for futile care, it won't be because this violates the patient's right to autonomy.

This account of the right to autonomy might be challenged, however, because it rests on a particular interpretation of the ideal of *respect* for autonomy. The account assumes that respect for a person's autonomy is nothing but respect for her freedom. But one might argue that one reason we respect her freedom is that we respect her moral *agency*—her unique ability to make the best choices for herself. If respect for autonomy is understood as respect for agency and not just respect for freedom, then a refusal to provide what the competent patient has requested might be seen as disrespectful of the patient's agency. This then would pose a direct conflict with the physician's duty of professional integrity.

So right off we have decisions to make about the interpretation and the justification of one of the initial principles, respect for autonomy. Our inquiry could just as well have turned toward the duty of professional integrity. We might ask what core values or precepts are integral to the responsible practice of medicine. Providing effective rather than ineffective care is certainly one. Avoiding pointlessly harmful "treatments" could be another. But how about incorporating patients' values and goals into plans of care? Not a traditional medical value, perhaps. But the more recent rhetoric of "patient-centered care" and "shared decision-making" suggests it may be one now. If acting on this value is also part of responsible medical practice, then all the ambiguities of "respect for autonomy" just discussed become a problem for determining what professional integrity itself requires in the face of patients' demands.

Our attempt to understand and justify the initial moral claim started with principles, and this in turn led to further questions about those principles, with answers framed in terms of yet other principles. We are trying to make a decision about the initial moral claim by seeing how it fits into a framework of principled commitments, hoping that the larger context will provide some decisive answer to the initial question. This effort to strike a wide reflective equilibrium will almost surely be a first step when trying to resolve serious disagreement about a claim of principle. For the reasons discussed in Chapter 2, however, this is not likely by itself to be sufficient. Other methods will need to come into play.

These could include appeals to paradigm cases. As noted above, there is a wealth of paradigm cases supporting the patient's right to refuse treatment, although the relevance of those cases for a duty to comply with patients' demands for treatment is in dispute. One can also put forward paradigm cases that support the physician's prerogative to say "no." Physicians should refuse to prescribe antibiotics for the common cold. Surgeons can refuse to operate on patients at high risk of dying during surgery. One might object that these so-called paradigms just beg the question by assuming that respect for patient autonomy doesn't trump professional integrity. This would drop us into the problem of deciding whether it is the principle or the considered judgment that carries the most probative weight—a question for which the method of reflective equilibrium is not well suited, as we've seen.

Another strategy might accept the paradigm cases of professional integrity as givens, and then see how morally similar they are to cases involving so-called futile treatment. One contrast might be this. Many of the paradigm cases of professional integrity withhold treatments with low stakes for the patient— for instance, because the patient will get better without the treatment he's demanding, like antibiotics for his cold. But the debate over medical futility is not about these kinds of cases. It's about cases in which the patient will most certainly die without the treatment he demands. Even if the chances of success are low, the stakes are the highest possible—the patient's last chance to live (Gampel, 2006). And so the claim of professional integrity won't warrant a decision to withhold high-stakes treatments like CPR if it's grounded in an appeal to such paradigm cases.

This foray into casuistical reasoning is relevant, certainly. But it may not get us very far, for some of the reasons found in the earlier discussion of casuistry. First, we can't be selective in our appeals to paradigm cases. Although refusing to prescribe antibiotics for a cold isn't very high stakes, refusing to take a patient to surgery can be. Then the question will be whether the surgeon's traditional prerogative has something to do with the magnitude of the harm she may inflict by her own hand. If the answer is "yes," then once it's pointed out that procedures like CPR are anything but harmless the question will be whether withholding futile CPR should be compared with the paradigm case of withholding antibiotics, or the paradigm case of refusing to take a patient to surgery. The problem is selecting which paradigm case or cases is the pertinent one. Addressing that question will take us back up into principles, even if the discussion of them will now be better informed by cases.

Evaluating a claim of principle will almost always entail interpretation of key concepts within it. In this case, of course, it's "futile," a concept that's spawned notions of physiological, quantitative, and qualitative futility (see Schneiderman, Jecker, and Jonson, 1990; Youngner, 1988). These are attempts to determine the legitimate scope of the principle—by determining when it's impossible for an intervention to produce any medical benefit, or the likelihood is too low to justify its use (physiological and quantitative futility); or by identifying types of benefit that patients and families are best able to judge (qualitative futility). Such conceptual distinctions are often undergirded by examples, and this opens up a role for narrative.

I vividly remember a story told to me by a physician after I'd given a talk on futility. She'd been caring for a patient with advanced HIV/AIDS, in the days before protease inhibitors had succeeded in making HIV a chronic disease for many. When his disease reached its terminal phase, with many body systems failing, the cardiac arrest that resulted could almost certainly not be reversed with CPR. Despite numerous discussions with him, he insisted that he remain a "full code" to the end, and made this a condition of his agreement to enter a hospice program. Perhaps he worried that having a DNR order would lead to neglect of his other needs, despite her reassurances to the contrary. His insistence presented her with a dilemma. On the one hand, there was every reason to believe that the resuscitation attempt would provide no medical benefit—that is, it would not prolong his life. But on the other, promising to make the futile attempt would secure his agreement to enter hospice, so that the quality of his remaining life would be as high as possible.

The story brought home to me the importance of recognizing that medical interventions have all kinds of effects besides the ones directly intended. There is no such thing as "futile," full stop. The question must always be, futile with respect to what goal? And when the goal being served is not one the physician had originally intended, the next question will be whether it is a goal that a responsible physician could or should serve by doing what has been asked.

We're unlikely to recognize such non-medical goals if we haven't talked with the patient or family enough to understand how a decision about "futile" treatment might reverberate in their lives. We need, in other words, to spin out that story. We need to do this not only to make a decision about a particular case. We may need also to confront the challenge to our understanding of "professional integrity" that the story's ending may present. Recognizing the necessity of this narrative exploration, and its implications, may reveal the danger of relying upon any fixed notion of "professional integrity." This is not a direct objection to the principle that physicians sometimes have the right to say "no" to protect their professional integrity. But it surely complicates what we take that principle to mean, and how we are to apply it in practice (see Tomlinson and Czlonka, 1995).

As our exploration of the debate about futile treatment has illustrated, a decision about a moral principle may well require more than appeal to other moral principles. It may need to pull in other methods as well, even those that might seem more suited to questions about cases, like casuistry or narrative. So far the methods aren't neatly aligning with the kind of moral problem, whether about a case or about a principle. Rather, the lesson is that we need to be attuned to the questions raised at various stages in the give-and-take of the argument, and be prepared to use whatever method fits the question.

Let's see if the lesson applies to decisions about policies as well.

Decisions About Practices and Policies

A decision about a practice or policy requires judgments of how to respond to a class of choices. Should we prohibit them entirely, permit them freely, or permit them subject to various restrictions or procedures? In contrast to a particular judgment about an individual case, a practice or policy deliberately establishes a rule or set of rules to be followed with regard to cases of a certain type. The behavior required by the rule may be at odds with at least some judgments made about individual cases of the type governed by the rule. Like a general moral principle, a policy can lead to judgments in individual cases that may not be warranted on other moral grounds. A decision that the policy is nonetheless justifiable requires the claim that on balance it is more likely than alternative policies to support good decisions rather than poor ones. Thus, there is always an implicit balancing judgment underlying any policy conclusion.

There is another important feature of practices or policies that distinguishes them from judgments about individual cases on the one hand, and general moral principles or rules on the other. That is the fact that they are promulgated and enacted by a group. This in turn places them into a different causal network that affects the range of consequences likely to be relevant to their moral evaluation. In evaluating a policy, one must account for how widely it is likely to be followed, what variety of interpretations are likely to be applied to it, the range of circumstances in which it is likely to be applied, and other aspects of the social environment in which the policy will play out. In comparison with the individual case, the web of consequences is much more complex, encompassing many more actors, dispersed in time and space.

Unlike questions about moral principle or rule, in questions of policy the consequences to be considered are not confined to the logical implications of the policy within a moral system that assesses how the policy *should* be understood and applied. Although this evaluation must be made, we must also contend with how the policy or rule *will* be understood and applied by those who use it.

Let's use as our illustrative example the claim that as a matter of social policy, economic incentives for organ donation should not be permitted. As before, the question throughout will be what this example can tell us about the usefulness of the various methods we've discussed in this book.

First, note that this claim needs to be put in the context of a set of principles, goals, or values taken to be central to the organ donation and transplantation *system*. As I just noted, the consequences of policies are always a product of the system in which they are implemented, and so it will be important to account for how the policy will affect the functionality of that system. In the case of organ transplantation, these would include such things as maximizing the availability of transplantable organs relative to need; avoiding unfairness in the distribution of organs; avoiding exploitation in the methods of procuring organs; respecting cultural values and taboos concerning treatment of the dead; expressing or protecting social values such as altruism; and potentially many others.

Thus, Arnold et al. (2002) argue against the use of direct financial payment for donation in part because it would undermine the centrality of altruism as the motivating value behind donation of organs. This argument illustrates two key tasks that need to be tackled when ethically evaluating any policy. One is to support the assumption that the value, goal, or principle being appealed to is in fact germane to the policy question, and the other is to show that it would either be threatened (or strengthened) under the policy alternative being proposed.

Regarding the first task, Arnold et al. take it as a virtual given that altruism should be the primary motivation for organ donation. But why should it be? Part of their answer is to suggest that the only alternative to altruism is "commoditization" of the body, and that this in turn has a variety of unsavory consequences, such as exploitation of the poor or manipulation of donors. Their object is to place the role of altruism in organ donation within the framework of a larger system of values. Here they would be arguing in the manner of a wide reflective equilibrium, showing how the insistence on altruism best serves this larger set of values. The arguments linking altruism to these other values would each need to be evaluated on its own terms, of course.

One would also need to consider arguments *challenging* the ideal of altruism in organ donation. So, for example, some have argued that cadaveric organ donation is a duty, since it sacrifices no significant interest of the dead, while serving the vital interests of the living (Nelson, 2003). In the fulfillment of duties, talk of altruism is out of place. Others argue that altruism is an instrumental value, to be preserved only insofar as it serves the more fundamental goal of securing transplantable organs. When some other motive better serves that goal, altruism should be sidelined. Still others, particularly feminists, have argued that the promotion of altruistic self-sacrifice is a dangerous business when it results in injustice or insensitivity to the significance of the harms suffered by those who make sacrifices, including organ donors or their families (Mongoven, 2003). These are arguments about the nature, desirability, and scope of altruism as a virtue.

As these differing arguments suggest, judgments about the relevance of a value, principle, or goal to the policy question will need to examine how it implicates other important values and beliefs when it is employed in the context in which the policy will be applied. This is an argument taking place at a relatively high level of generality, making it seem unlikely that more particular methods, like narrative and casuistry, will find a use. That would be a hasty conclusion, as we will see in a moment.

After considering the relevance of the value or principle being employed, the next key task is to explain how the alternatives being considered for policy each implicate the value in question. And so, the burden on those opposed to the use of financial incentives is to show that such incentives are incompatible— necessarily, or contingently—with preserving the idea that the donation is an altruistic gift.

Some may argue they are not necessarily incompatible, so long as the incentive only lowers the barriers to acting altruistically, and is not by itself a sufficient motive. Tax deductions for donations to charities encourage people to donate, but since the donation remains a net loss, it is still a sacrifice motivated at least in part by altruism, and so it is still properly called a donation. Self-interested and altruistic reasons can sometimes operate alongside one another (Tomlinson, 1992). If tax deductions for charitable donations serve as a paradigm case of this possibility, it invites a casuistical argument: which incentives for organ donation, if any, are comparable to tax deductions? Here, then, we have one likely entry point for the casuistical method in policy debates: helping to determine whether, by its nature, the policy option under consideration is consistent with some already agreed-upon governing principle, value, or goal.

If incentives are not necessarily incompatible with altruism, then the task will be to show that *particular kinds* of incentive are incompatible. So, when Arnold et al. (2002) consider the variety of forms that inducements might take, they claim that while a tax credit is a form of payment inconsistent with altruism, reimbursement of funeral expenses or a donation to a charity in the donor's name doesn't threaten this fundamental value (so long as the reimbursement or donation is not too large). They provide very little explanation of this distinction. The distinction begs for an argument, in light of the observation above concerning tax deductions for charitable donations. One might wonder, for example, what the difference is between a tax credit (which like a deduction results in a savings on taxes paid) and a reimbursement of funeral expenses (which also results in a savings, this time on funeral costs paid).

There are two ways to continue the argument on a question like this. One is to go on with the casuistical analysis that we've started, in an attempt to show whether the acceptance of that form of payment exemplifies non-altruistic behavior by its very nature.

The other is to provide evidence that a particular option (in this case, a particular form of incentive) *in fact* would erode the value in question. One sort of argument would rely on psychological or sociological theories and evidence showing how a particular option would lead to or encourage behavior or attitudes clearly contrary to the value in question. But another alternative is to turn to more personal stories that persuasively illustrate some recognizably human difficulty in maintaining altruistic motives alongside economic incentives. It wouldn't matter whether these were "real-life" accounts, or fictional. The criterion of evaluation would be their verisimilitude. Do the stories resonate with what we know of human motives, feelings, relationships, and decisions? Or are they ginned-up morality tales constructed to serve a fixed conclusion? Since the question of how people will employ or respond to a policy option is obviously of critical importance, narratives may often have a role to play in policy debates.

So in our brief discussion of this one policy question, we've identified ways in which principles within a reflective equilibrium, casuistry, virtues, and narrative might be brought to bear. As with the other contexts we've examined, these are not methods in competition with one another over the same task. As before, debates over the principles, goals, or values at stake set a framework within which other methods find a problem to solve. In this case, casuistry helps to determine whether economic incentives are necessarily at odds with the virtue of altruism, and narrative offers one way to evaluate whether altruism would be undermined as a matter of fact. Such questions presuppose a principled commitment to maintaining altruism as a primary motive within organ donation.

Summing Up

As these examples have demonstrated, different methods don't line up neatly behind particular types of ethical problem. Instead, various methods play different *roles* within the course of reasoned deliberation. Although the initial structure of the problem may often be set by the moral principles in contention, the deliberation that follows may need to use any of the methods we've discussed in the book. Which of them are used will depend on the paths taken in the give-and-take of argument over a problem, and the types of question raised by that argument. This calls for an imaginative flexibility in our understanding and use of these methods that's capable of seeing the opportunity to employ one method or another at the right juncture. This requires a keen appreciation of the nature of each of these methods, and of their characteristic strengths and weaknesses—the focus of this book. Development of that appreciation, and the capacity to use it appropriately and creatively, comes only with practice—something no book can provide.

Note

1 The Committee actually excused their decision on a technicality: the center had in place a standard practice not to accept sperm donation from men above a certain age, and so Irene's father was disqualified on those grounds. Thus it avoided having to explain the moral basis of its decision, which was in fact motivated by other concerns.

Bibliography

Arnold, Robert, et al. 2002. "Financial Incentives for Cadaver Organ Donation: An Ethical Reappraisal." *Transplantation* 73(8): 1361–1367.

Forrow, Lachlan. 2002a. "An Ethicist's View." *Journal of Clinical Ethics* 13(3):233, 240.

Forrow, Lachlan. 2002b. "Moving from Moral Judgment to Ethical Reasoning." *Journal of Clinical Ethics* 13(3):234, 242–246.

Gampel, Eric. 2006. "Does Professional Autonomy Protect Medical Futility Judgments?" *Bioethics* 20(2):92–104.

High, Dallas M. 1988. "All in the Family: Extended Autonomy and Expectations in Surrogate Health Care Decision-Making." *Gerontologist* 128(3 Suppl):46–51.

Klipstein, Sigal. 2002a. "Irene's View." *Journal of Clinical Ethics* 13(3): 232, 235–237.

Klipstein, Sigal. 2002b. "Irene's Physician's View." *Journal of Clinical Ethics* 13(3):232, 237.

Klipstein, Sigal. 2002c. "New Reproductive Options and the Incest Taboo." *Journal of Clinical Ethics* 13(3):234, 240–241.

Mongoven, Ann. 2003. "Sharing Our Body and Blood: Organ Donation and Feminist Critiques of Sacrifice." *Journal of Medicine and Philosophy* 28(1):89–114.

Nelson, James L. 2003. "A Duty to Donate? Selves, Societies, and Organ Procurement." In James L. Nelson. *Hippocrates' Maze: Ethical Explorations of the Medical Labyrinth.* New York: Rowan and Littlefield.

O'Neill, Stephen. 2002. "The Social Worker's View." *Journal of Clinical Ethics* 13(3):233, 238–239.

Schneiderman, Lawrence J., Nancy S. Jecker, and Albert R. Jonsen. 1990. "Medical Futility: Its Meaning and Ethical Implications." *Annals of Internal Medicine* 112(12):949–954.

Tomlinson. Tom. 1992. "Inducements for Donation: Benign Incentives or Risky Business?" *Transplantation Proceedings* 24(5):2204–2206.

Tomlinson, Tom. 2001. "Futile Care in Oncology: When to Stop Trying", *The Lancet Oncology* 2:759–761.

Tomlinson, Tom. 2007. "Futility beyond CPR: The Case of Dialysis." *HEC (Healthcare Ethics Committee) Forum* 19(1):33–43.

Tomlinson, Tom, and Howard Brody. 1990. "Futility and the Ethics of Resuscitation." *JAMA* 264(10):1276–1280.

Tomlinson, Tom, and Diane Czlonka. 1995. "Futility and Hospital Policy." *Hastings Center Report* 25(3):28–35.

Tomlinson, Tom, Kenneth Howe, Mark Notman, and Diane Rossmiller. 1990. "An Empirical Study of Proxy Consent for the Elderly." *The Gerontologist* 30:54–64.

Tovey, Philip. 1998. "Narrative Knowledge Development in Medical Ethics." *Journal of Medical Ethics* 24:176–181.

Youngner, Stuart J. 1988. "Who Defines Futility?" *JAMA* 260(14): 2094–2095.

INDEX

Abelard, Peter, 201
abortion, 31–35
  analogical reasoning for, 107–8
  Christian attitudes and, 32
  conception of property and, 44n11
  feminist medical ethics and, 159–60
  fetus potentiality and, 31–32
  preference utilitarianism and, 34
  prior existence principles for, 33
  secular morality and, 37
  theory of the good and, 40
  virtue theory and, 201
The Abuse of Casuistry (Jonsen/Toulmin), 84
accidental killing, 210n8
acquired immunodeficiency syndrome (AIDS), 206–9
active euthanasia, 17
  casuistry and, 101
  DDE and, 203
advance directives, 133

affective-receptive interaction, in ethics of care, 177
age-based allocation, 81n16
aggregate utility, 44n7
AIDS. *See* acquired immunodeficiency syndrome
Allmark, Peter, 178
Alsop, Stuart, 132
altruism
  economic incentives and, 233
  as medical practice and policy, 231–32
  as virtue, 207
American Medical Association, 17
analogical reasoning
  for abortion, 107–8
  in casuistry, xiii, 88, 103
  ethical reasoning through, 112n3
  paradigm cases and, 106
  principle testing for, 109–11
  social consequence assessment from, 107–8
applied ethics, circular reasoning and, 27